A Balanced Approach to

PCOS

16 Weeks of Meal Prep & Recipes for Women Managing Polycystic Ovary Syndrome

MELISSA GROVES AZZARO, RDN, LD

VICTORY BELT PUBLISHING INC.

LAS VEGAS

First published in 2020 by Victory Belt Publishing Inc.

Copyright © 2020 Melissa Groves Azzaro, RDN, LD

ISBN-13: 978-1-628604-13-9

The information included in this book is for educational purposes only. It is not intended or implied to be a substitute for professional medical advice. The reader should consult her healthcare provider to determine the appropriateness of the information for her own situation or if she has any questions regarding a medical condition or treatment plan.

Cover design by Justin-Aaron Velasco

Interior design and illustrations by Crizalie Olimpo, Charisse Reyes, Elita San Juan, and Allan Santos

Photos of author by Alexis the Greek Digital Media LLC

Printed in Canada

TC 0222

To my late grandmother, Grace Mulligan, for being my first cooking teacher through example. Many times during the development of this book, I found myself comparing myself to my memories of you in the kitchen. And in my memories, you were always in the kitchen. Thank you for teaching me the irreplaceable value of quality ingredients and that cooking for someone is a perfectly acceptable way of demonstrating your love for them.

Table of **CONTENTS**

ACKNOWLEDGMENTS

There are so many people in my life without whom this book would not be possible. I am deeply grateful for every single person who has, in some way great or small, helped me along my journey to create a successful business as a second career as a dietitian and bring this book to fruition.

First, always, and forever, my husband, Matt Azzaro, for supporting me in more ways than I can count, from being my first taster (and losing weight after months of following the PCOS diet plan!), to washing literal tons of dishes, to keeping the rest of our world running and caring for our furs (Artie, Max, Olivia, and Skeeter) for months, to providing emotional support when I was essentially working three full-time jobs simultaneously. I truly could not do what I do without his support.

My family, Ellen and Michael Groves and Carmela and Sam Azzaro, who provided unconditional love and support and have always been supportive of my efforts in the kitchen. Special thanks to my English major aunt, Chris Mulligan, for encouraging my writing from an early age.

My friends and colleagues who supported me along the way. Special shout-outs to loyal friends Heather Snyder Ippolito, Shelby Guptill, Sue St. Martin, and Erin Allgood. And to RD colleagues Elizabeth Shaw, Lauren Manaker, Kendra Tolbert, Kristin Willard, Christine Dyan, Martha McKittrick, Cory Levin, Tamara Melton, and the entire board of the Dietitians in Integrative and Functional Medicine Dietetic Practice Group of the Academy of Nutrition and Dietetics—you inspire me every day with the work you are doing. A special thank you to Maxine Mallawaarachchi for her assistance with the development of materials for my course, The PCOS Root Cause Roadmap, which was launching for the first time simultaneously with the writing of this book.

Thank you to Alexis the Greek for author photography and to all the locations that allowed us to take photos in their beautiful spaces, especially Shelby and Conor Guptill for the use of their sunny kitchen and Tendercrop Farm at the Red Barn in Dover, New Hampshire. Thanks also to Shaw's Supermarket in North Hampton, New Hampshire, especially the seafood department, for always providing me with perfectly cut fillets.

I would also like to thank all my former professors and preceptors who encouraged me to keep going, especially Dr. Collette Janson-Sand, Lance Westergard, and my culinary skills professors.

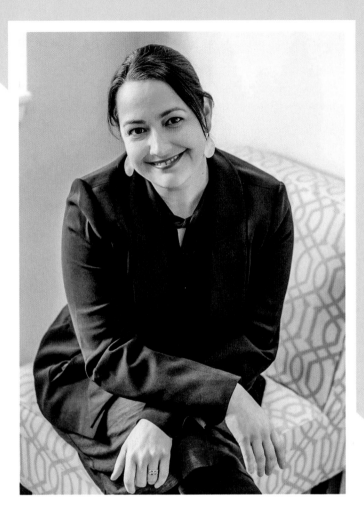

Thank you to the whole team at Victory Belt. I have felt so cared for throughout this process, especially as a first-time author.

Finally, thank you to all the women who have trusted me in their journeys to gain control over their hormones and fertility, whether as one-on-one clients, as students of my courses, or as part of my online world. You are the reason I do what I do. Every time I get a message that one of you has gotten your period without medication, has had a positive pregnancy test, or has brought a baby into this world, I know how important it is for me to keep going, because the work I'm doing truly matters. Thank you.

INTRODUCTION

Nine years ago, I was sitting in the living room of my Brooklyn apartment when I had a breakthrough.

I had just worked an eighty-plus-hour week; back then, I worked as an advertising copywriter, and I was extremely good at my job. My company often used my talent as an excuse to overwork me, though I used to feel that all the extra hours I put in, the extensive travel, and the ignoring of everything else in my life—including the food I put in my body—were marks of success. This fateful night, I was about to place my usual "healthy takeout" order (because I'd traveled out of the country earlier in the week and literally had no food in the fridge) when I realized I'd had enough. I was tired of compromising my health for my job.

Sure, I had developed all sorts of strategies and shortcuts for feeding myself as well as I could manage, but the truth was, I was spending a lot of money on takeout, I didn't have time to exercise (I'd just had to bail on running the New York City Marathon for the third year in a row), and I was drinking far too much coffee in the morning to get going and far too much wine at night to wind down.

Something had to change. I needed an escape plan—and fast.

That's when I experienced one of those "duh" moments. I realized that I had all the tools I needed at my disposal; I just needed to commit myself to a new plan. I started reading nutrition and health books, cookbooks, and food politics books. I began to pay attention to what my body was actually asking for and stopped forcing it to accept whatever I had time to give it. I quit my job, realizing that my "successes" at work were causing me more harm than good.

In short, I chose my health.

After a long period of study, I decided to become a dietitian to help others experiencing burnout regain control over their lives.

I got interested in women's health and hormones in my first job as a registered dietitian in the office of a functional medicine practitioner. I saw all the clients who wanted to focus on weight loss. I would review their diet and exercise routines and couldn't see why these women weren't losing weight. Calories in, calories out, right? But since functional medicine uses a root-cause approach, I dug a little deeper, and what I found was that almost all of these women were suffering from a hormone imbalance of some kind, whether it was high insulin or insulin resistance, high cortisol, low thyroid hormone, or a condition such as polycystic ovary syndrome (PCOS), in which levels of androgen (male hormones) are higher than they should be.

It felt like a light bulb had gone off. What if we approached diet by focusing on *balancing hormones* instead of losing weight? Weight is merely a *symptom* of unbalanced hormones. Balance the hormones and the weight comes to a healthy level naturally!

When I opened my own practice, I knew that I wanted to help women learn how to make diet and lifestyle changes that would balance their hormones so that they could have more energy, fewer cravings, and fewer hormonal symptoms like painful, heavy periods on one end of the spectrum or lack of ovulation and periods (such as with PCOS) on the other. Furthermore, I wanted to help women whose lives were like mine had been—who had the desire to eat well and the knowledge that good nutrition improves all aspects of their lives but lacked the time and energy to do what it takes.

I've now seen hundreds of women with PCOS, fertility issues, and other hormonal imbalances in my practice in person on the New Hampshire seacoast and virtually throughout the United States. And time and time again, I've seen how much of a difference nutrition makes in the lives of women with PCOS—from regaining their periods to losing weight naturally while eating more food than they ever have before, and even getting pregnant after years of trying.

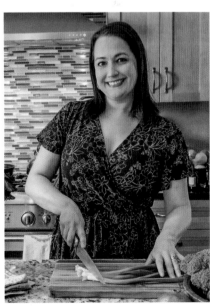

The key to success is a way of eating that addresses the root causes of PCOS. Even more importantly, it can be done with little time investment—just a bit of prep time will ensure that you'll eat well all week. Finally, the way of eating I recommend for PCOS is nonrestrictive: it doesn't eliminate any foods or food groups. PCOS is a lifelong condition; therefore, the way of eating you adopt should be sustainable for a lifetime.

I hope that this book helps you finally feel like you can gain control over your PCOS symptoms while eating meals that are as delicious as they are balanced. I believe in you, cyster!

To balanced hormones!

Melissa Groves Azzaro, RDN, LD

A Brief Overview of **PCOS**

If you've been diagnosed with polycystic ovary syndrome (PCOS), then you should know that it's not just about your ovaries. It is a complicated disorder that affects nearly every system of the body, including sex hormones, stress hormones, metabolism, and gut health.[1] It is estimated to affect 5 to 15 percent of women.[2] So you are not alone!

You should not take being diagnosed with PCOS lightly, because the disorder puts you at increased risk for infertility, diabetes, heart disease, obesity, and certain gynecological cancers.[3] The good news is that many of these risks can be reduced with diet and lifestyle.

HOW IS PCOS DIAGNOSED?

The most common way that PCOS is diagnosed is using the Rotterdam Criteria. According to these criteria, a woman must have two of the following three signs and symptoms[4]:

- Irregular or no ovulation
- High androgen (male hormone) levels detected on lab tests, or symptoms of high androgens, such as acne, facial hair, and male-pattern hair loss
- Multiple immature follicles ("cysts") on the ovaries

SYMPTOMS OF PCOS

There are several "types" of PCOS, and each woman experiences different symptoms, but some of the most common symptoms are[5]

- Acne
- Anxiety and depression
- Darkening of the skin or skin tags around the neck and armpits
- Difficulty getting pregnant
- Difficulty losing weight, especially in the belly area
- Disordered eating (especially binge eating disorder)
- Fatigue

- High blood sugar or insulin levels

- Hirsutism (excess hair growth on the face and body)

- Irregular ovulation and/or periods

- Strong cravings for carbs and sugar

- Thinning scalp hair

Targeting the Root Causes of PCOS:
THE PROTEIN + FAT + FIBER METHOD

Conventional medical treatment for PCOS focuses on treating symptoms with medications such as the birth control pill and fertility drugs.[6] In my practice, however, I use a functional medicine approach, meaning that I focus on addressing the underlying *causes* of the symptoms rather than on the symptoms themselves.

There are four root causes of PCOS:

PCOS ROOT CAUSES

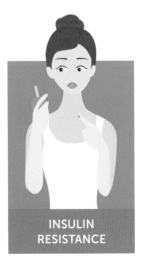
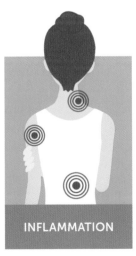
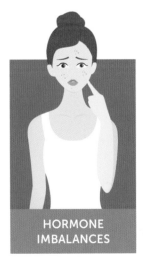
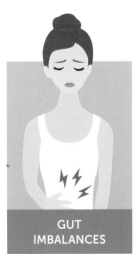

INSULIN RESISTANCE   INFLAMMATION   HORMONE IMBALANCES   GUT IMBALANCES

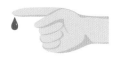

INSULIN RESISTANCE

Insulin resistance occurs when your cells stop responding to the insulin signal to let in glucose, leading to high sugar in your blood and low sugar inside your cells. Insulin resistance is common in women with PCOS, occurring in 75 percent of those who are of normal weight and 95 percent of those who are overweight.[7] It leads to higher circulating levels of insulin, which causes the ovaries to produce more testosterone (a type of androgen), making PCOS symptoms worse.[8]

HORMONE IMBALANCES

Hormone imbalances are common in PCOS, with the most common being higher-than-normal levels of androgens such as testosterone, DHEA, and DHT. However, PCOS also affects many of the hormones produced by the pituitary gland, ovaries, and adrenal glands.[11] Women with PCOS can have high or low estrogens, and progesterone is low due to lack of ovulation. Luteinizing hormone (LH) is often high as the body is trying to ovulate, and anti-Mullerian hormone (AMH) is high due to the high number of immature follicles within the ovaries. High testosterone levels interfere with normal ovulation, leading to irregular periods, and low progesterone (which becomes low due to lack of ovulation) raises the risk for cancers of the uterus.[12]

INFLAMMATION

Inflammation is a complicated process by which the body releases inflammatory compounds. Studies have shown that women with PCOS have higher levels of these compounds than women without PCOS.[9] Inflammation is an independent risk factor for heart disease and believed to be one of the reasons women with PCOS are at higher risk for heart disease and stroke. To make matters worse, obesity worsens inflammation.[10] So, if you have PCOS and you are overweight, chances are pretty good that you've also got some degree of inflammation present.

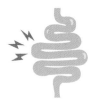

GUT IMBALANCES

You may be surprised to learn that gastrointestinal symptoms like bloating, constipation, and diarrhea are linked to PCOS. In one study, women with PCOS were more than four times more likely to have irritable bowel syndrome (IBS) than women without PCOS.[13] In another study, the bacteria found in the digestive tracts of women with PCOS were found to be different and less diverse than those in women who did not have the condition.[14] These changes in the gut microbiome can lead to higher androgen levels and androgen symptoms in women with PCOS.[15]

To effectively manage the symptoms of PCOS, you should follow a diet that targets insulin resistance, inflammation, hormone imbalances, and gut imbalances. An ideal diet for PCOS is one that is

- **Blood sugar balancing:** High in protein and moderate in carbohydrates
- **Anti-inflammatory:** High in colorful fruits and vegetables and healthy fats
- **Hormone balancing:** Incorporating hormone-balancing foods such as flaxseed and spearmint tea
- **Gut health supporting:** Including a variety of plant fibers to support beneficial bacteria growth as well as probiotics from fermented foods

For a diet to accomplish these four goals, it needs to include a balance of protein, fat, and fiber. I also recommend including what I've termed PCOS Power Foods, which are particularly helpful for PCOS.

ESSENTIAL COMPONENTS OF A PCOS MEAL PLAN

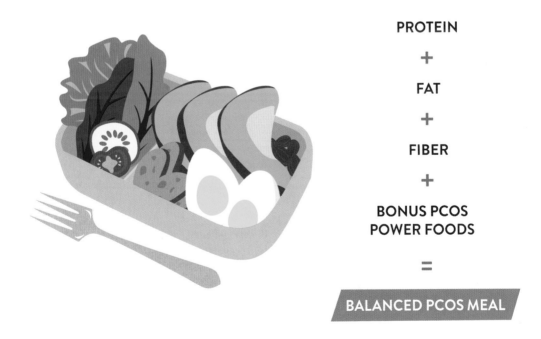

PROTEIN

+

FAT

+

FIBER

+

BONUS PCOS
POWER FOODS

=

BALANCED PCOS MEAL

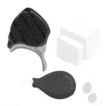

PROTEIN

Protein is beneficial for women with PCOS because it fills you up without raising your blood sugar. All of the meals in this book have been designed to include 25 to 30 grams of protein per serving, and all of the snacks/desserts have been designed to include 8 to 10 grams of protein.

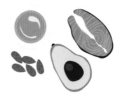

FAT

Fat also helps fill you up without raising your blood sugar—and it makes food taste good! The recipes in this book emphasize healthy fats such as those found in olive oil, nuts, avocados, and fatty fish. Aim to include 1 to 2 tablespoons of fat with each of your meals (10 to 20 grams per day).

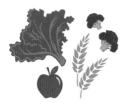

FIBER

Fiber helps slow the rate at which glucose enters your bloodstream after a meal. Additionally, it helps "feed" the good bacteria in your gut to keep your digestive system healthy and happy. Fiber is found in fruits, vegetables, legumes, and whole grains. Aim to include 30 to 35 grams a day, which breaks down to 7 to 10 grams per meal, plus at least a couple of grams from snacks.

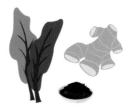

BONUS: PCOS POWER FOODS

Think of these as superfoods just for women with PCOS! They support PCOS by addressing at least one of the root causes listed above. These foods are optional, but the more you can work them into your diet, the better. I've included at least one of them in each week's menu in this book.

PCOS-FRIENDLY MEAL PLANNING

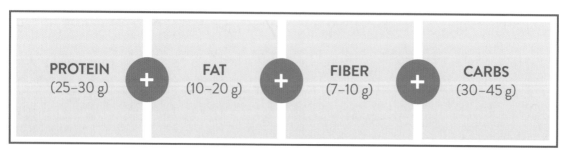

PROTEIN (25–30 g) + FAT (10–20 g) + FIBER (7–10 g) + CARBS (30–45 g)

A Balanced PCOS PLATE

So why don't I include carbs in the perfect PCOS plate? I always tell my clients that they don't have to work to include carbs—because carbs are everywhere.

When it comes to carbs, I have one "rule":

Never eat carbs by themselves.

OR—a different way of looking at it:

Always combine carbs with protein, fat, and fiber.

What does that look like in real life? Using the plate model, aim to make half of your plate nonstarchy, colorful veggies, at *least* one-quarter of your plate protein, and *no more than* one-quarter of your plate starchy carbs, and then add 1 to 2 tablespoons of fat.

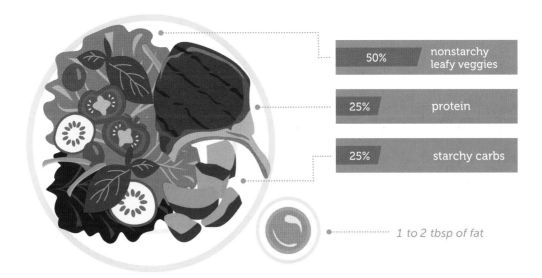

50% nonstarchy leafy veggies

25% protein

25% starchy carbs

1 to 2 tbsp of fat

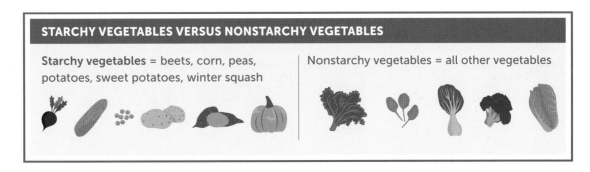

STARCHY VEGETABLES VERSUS NONSTARCHY VEGETABLES

Starchy vegetables = beets, corn, peas, potatoes, sweet potatoes, winter squash

Nonstarchy vegetables = all other vegetables

WHICH FOODS COUNT AS STARCHY CARBS?

 Grains (barley, quinoa, rice, wheat, etc.)

 Legumes (black beans, chickpeas, lentils, white beans, etc.)

 Processed grains (breads, cereals, pasta, pastries, etc.)

 Starchy veggies (see above)

A WORD ABOUT CARBOHYDRATE TOLERANCE

Carbohydrate needs vary from person to person depending on weight, activity level, degree of insulin resistance, and other factors. You may need more carbs than another woman with PCOS does. Alternatively, you might feel better if you eat fewer carbs.

I recommend starting with the amount of carbs/starches called for in the recipes in this book—approximately ½ cup per serving—and then adjusting upward or downward as needed.

Similarly, you may want to play around with carb timing. Experiment with having more or less carbs at different meals. Some women feel great including carbs with breakfast and lunch, but it makes others feel sluggish and tired. Some women feel better with a lower-carb dinner, while others don't really feel "full" and aren't able to sleep if they haven't had enough carbs in the evening meal. It's completely individual!

Why I Use a Nonrestrictive Approach to **PCOS**

There are many "PCOS diets" on the internet that include long laundry lists of foods you should "never" eat. These forbidden foods usually include carbs, sugar, dairy, gluten, "processed" foods, and more. Additionally, many people proclaim that a 100 percent plant-based diet is the key to PCOS, while just as many recommend ketogenic diets, which often include a lot of fatty meats and a low intake of fruits and vegetables.

I don't agree with these approaches for a few reasons:

- There's little to no evidence behind any of these recommendations:
  a. Zero studies on PCOS and gluten
  b. One study on PCOS and a dairy-free diet (which was also low in starch)[16]
  c. One study on PCOS and keto, and it involved eleven women, more than half of whom dropped out of the study before six months[17]

- Women with PCOS are at a significantly higher risk for eating disorders, especially binge eating disorder.[18] One of the biggest triggers for episodes of bingeing is a restrictive diet.

- I believe that there is room for all foods in a healthy diet—it's how you balance them that matters. (Add that protein, fat, and fiber!)

- PCOS is a lifelong condition; therefore, any dietary changes made should be sustainable for a lifetime.

A WORD ABOUT TREATS

Similarly, I believe that there is room for treats in any healthy diet. Just because you've been diagnosed with PCOS doesn't mean you're never allowed to eat a cookie or a piece of birthday cake again!

So I've included a few treats in the Supplemental Recipes section of this book. To minimize the effects of sweet treats on blood sugar balance, here are a few tricks:

- Eat them as soon after a balanced meal as possible.
- Combine them with protein (such as Greek yogurt or protein powder), fat (such as nuts), and fiber (such as fruit).
- Boost dessert recipes you love by adding protein, fat, and fiber to improve their nutrient profile.

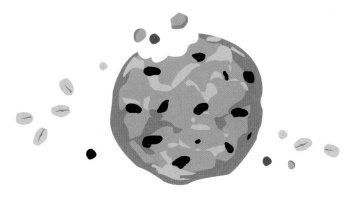

Will the Recipes in This Book
HELP ME LOSE WEIGHT?

I wouldn't be a very good dietitian if I didn't answer that question with, "It depends!" Theoretically, if you're balancing your hormones by eating this way, then your weight should start to come into balance. In my practice, we don't focus on the scale. Instead, we focus on building sustainable healthy behaviors, such as meal prep. Using this book is a great way to get in the habit of making that happen.

So let's get started!

REFERENCES

1. H. Teede, A. Deeks, and L. Moran, "Polycystic ovary syndrome: a complex condition with psychological, reproductive and metabolic manifestations that impacts on health across the lifespan," *BMC Medicine 8* (2010): 41, doi:10.1186/1741-7015-8-41.

2. D. A. Dumesic, S. E. Oberfield, E. Stener-Victorin, J. C. Marshall, J. S. Laven, and R. S. Legro, "Scientific statement on the diagnostic criteria, epidemiology, pathophysiology, and molecular genetics of polycystic ovary syndrome," *Endocrine Reviews* 36, no. 5 (2015): 487–525, doi:10.1210/er.2015-1018.

3. L. C. Torchen, "Cardiometabolic risk in PCOS: more than a reproductive disorder," *Current Diabetes Reports* 17, no. 12 (2017): 137, doi:10.1007/s11892-017-0956-2; E. Diamani-Kandarakis and A. Dunaif, "Insulin resistance and the polycystic ovary syndrome revisited: an update on mechanisms and implications," *Endocrine Reviews* 33, no. 6 (2012): 981–1030, doi:10.1210/er.2011-1034.

4. Rotterdam ESHRE/ASRM-sponsored PCOS consensus workshop group 2004, Revised 2003 consensus on diagnostic criteria and long-term health risks related to polycystic ovary syndrome, *Fertility and Sterility* 81: 19–25, doi:10.1016/j.fertnstert.2003.10.004.

5. International evidence-based guideline for the assessment and management of polycystic ovary syndrome, 2018, Monash University, Melbourne, Australia, ISBN-13: 978-0-646-98332-5.

6. J. Y. Oh, H. Lee, J. Y. Oh, Y. A. Sung, and H. Chung, "Serum C-reactive protein levels in normal-weight polycystic ovary syndrome," *Korean Journal of Internal Medicine* 24, no. 4 (2009): 350–55, doi:10.3904/kjim.2009.24.4.350.

7. See note 5 above.

8. Torchen, "Cardiometabolic risk in PCOS" (see note 3 above).

9. See note 6 above.

10. M. S. Ellulu, I. Patimah, H. Khaza'ai, A. Rahmat, and Y. Abed, "Obesity and inflammation: the linking mechanism and the complications," *Archives of Medical Science* 13, no. 4 (2017): 851–63, doi:10.5114/aoms.2016.58928.

11. R. L. Rosenfield and D. A. Ehrmann, "The pathogenesis of polycystic ovary syndrome (PCOS): The hypothesis of PCOS as functional ovarian hyperandrogenism revisited," *Endocrine Reviews* 37, no. 5 (2016): 467–520, doi:10.1210/er.2015-1104 .

12. J. A. Barry, M. M. Azizia, and P. J. Hardiman, "Risk of endometrial, ovarian and breast cancer in women with polycystic ovary syndrome: a systematic review and meta-analysis," *Human Reproduction Update* 20, no. 5 (2014): 748–58, doi:10.1093/humupd/dmu012.

13. R. Mathur, A. Ko, L. G. Hwang, K. Low, R. Azziz, and M. Pimentel, "Polycystic ovary syndrome is associated with an increased prevalence of irritable bowel syndrome," *Digestive Diseases and Sciences* 55 (2010): 1085–89, doi:10.1007/s10620-009-0890-5.

14. L. Lindheim, M. Bashir, J. Münzker, et al., "Alterations in gut microbiome composition and barrier function are associated with reproductive and metabolic defects in women with polycystic ovary syndrome (PCOS): A pilot study," *PLoS One* 12, no. 1 (2017): e0168390, doi:10.1371/journal.pone.0168390.

15. P. J. Torres, M. Siakowska, B. Banaszewska, et al., "Gut microbial diversity in women with polycystic ovary syndrome correlates with hyperandrogenism," *Journal of Clinical Endocrinology and Metabolism* 103, no. 4 (2018): 1502–11, doi:10.1210/jc.2017-02153.

16. J. L. Phy, A. M. Pohlmeier, J. A. Cooper, et al., "Low starch / low dairy diet results in successful treatment of obesity and co-morbidities linked to polycystic ovary syndrome (PCOS)," *Journal of Obesity and Weight Loss Therapy* 5, no. 2 (2015): 259, doi:10.4172/2165-7904.1000259.

17. J. C. Mavropoulos, W. S. Yancy, J. Hepburn, and E. C. Westman, "The effects of a low-carbohydrate, ketogenic diet on the polycystic ovary syndrome: a pilot study," *Nutrition & Metabolism* (London) 2 (2005): 35, doi:10.1186/1743-7075-2-35.

18. I. Lee, L. G. Cooney, S. Saini, M. E. Smith, M. D. Sammel, K. C. Allison, and A. Dokras, "Increased risk of disordered eating in polycystic ovary syndrome," *Fertility and Sterility* 107, no. 3 (2017): 796–802, doi: 10.1016/j.fertnstert.2016.12.014.

Using This BOOK

This book is organized by season (winter, spring, summer, and fall), with four weeks' worth of meal plans for each season featuring seasonal ingredients and flavors.

Each week includes recipes for two breakfasts, two lunches, and two dinners using a featured protein, fat, fiber, and PCOS Power Food (see page 14). Feel free to mix and match them as you like or make them all!

Most of the recipes in these plans make two servings, with the exception of the muffin recipes, which make more. You can adjust the quantities up or down depending on the number of people you're feeding.

For other meals that aren't covered by the plans, follow the Protein + Fat + Fiber method (see pages 11 to 14) to ensure that you're keeping your blood sugar balanced. This method works no matter where you are—whether you're in a restaurant, traveling, or even eating takeout.

You can also supplement the meal plans as needed with the balanced smoothies and snacks that appear in the Supplemental Recipes section of this book, beginning on page 289. Additionally, I have included healthy dessert recipes for those occasions when you need a healthier option. These are not intended to be included every day or week.

STEP 1: CHOOSE A WEEK.

When choosing which week you'd like to make, consider the following:

- Does it feature any ingredients that you don't like or aren't currently available in your area?

- Do these dishes meet your nutrition needs? See the section "Customizing Meals" (pages 24 to 25) to adjust the recipes to meet any dietary restrictions you may have. Note that for each week, I have included simple instructions for adding more carbs and for making the meals dairy-free.

Once you've chosen the week you want to make, determine the number of servings to make based on your needs. Are you feeding just one or two people, or are you feeding a family?

STEP 2: SHOP FOR FOOD.

- Use the Weekly Ingredients list to make a list of what you'll need at the store. The list assumes that you'll be making all six recipes for the week. Make sure to adjust the ingredient quantities if you scale the recipes up or down to make more or less food.

- Check to see what you already have in your fridge, freezer, and pantry before you go shopping.

STEP 3: PREP MEAL COMPONENTS IN ADVANCE.

Each week includes a Prep Day, on which you'll do some of the prep work to save yourself time in the kitchen during the week. This includes chopping and roasting vegetables and precooking grains, starches, and proteins.

I've recommended the cooking methods that I like and use most, but if you have access to an Instant Pot, a slow cooker, or another appliance you prefer using, feel free to use that instead.

STEP 4: MAKE THE RECIPES AS YOU GO.

When you are ready to make one of the meals, refer to the recipe in the Recipes section for the week. Use your already prepped and cooked components, which are marked with check marks in the ingredient lists, to make the meals. With so much of the prep work already done, the aim is for weekday cooking to be as quick as possible.

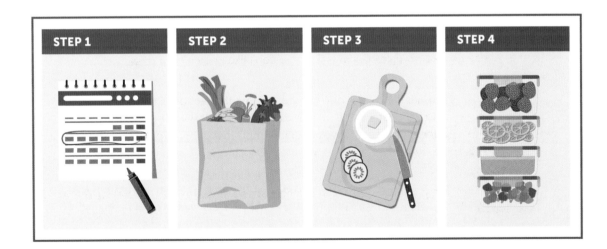

INGREDIENTS USED IN THIS BOOK

There are some ingredients used within the recipes in this book that you may not be familiar with, but that have benefits for women with PCOS. Here is a quick overview of what they are and where you can find them:

BONE BROTH

Bone broth is one of those "trendy" ingredients for good reason: it contains far more protein than normal beef or chicken stock. Using bone broth as the base for a soup gives it a protein boost, but if you can't find it, you can substitute beef or chicken stock.

COLLAGEN PEPTIDES

Hydrolyzed beef collagen is a flavorless powder that adds amino acids (protein) to recipes without altering the flavor. If you don't eat meat but do eat fish, you may substitute marine collagen. There are no vegetarian sources of collagen, but you may substitute a plant-based protein powder such as pea protein if you prefer.

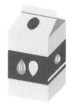

NONDAIRY MILKS

Nondairy milks are milk substitutes that are widely available in grocery stores. When selecting a nondairy milk to use in a recipe, consider the flavor (coconut milk has a stronger flavor than almond milk, for example), as well as the nutrient profile. Coconut milk is higher in fat but lower in carbs; rice milk and oat milk, on the other hand, are mostly carbs. Most nondairy milks are low in protein; however, soy milk has around the same protein content as dairy milk, and there are some pea protein–based milks that can add protein without changing the flavor of a recipe too much. Regardless of the type you choose, be sure to select one that is unsweetened to avoid added sugar.

NUT BUTTERS

I recommend several nut and seed butters throughout the recipes in this book. Peanut butter is fine to use if more expensive nut butters such as almond and cashew are outside of your budget. Sunflower seed butter is a great alternative made from seeds, which makes it a good option for those with nut allergies. Look for nut butters without added sweeteners. If it's important for you to use a smooth variety in a particular recipe in order to get the right texture, I'll note that in the ingredient list.

PROTEIN POWDER

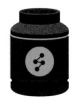

I recommend finding an unflavored protein powder with as few added ingredients as possible and no added sugars or artificial sweeteners. A protein powder that is pure protein is going to add protein to a recipe without changing its flavor. Feel free to use whey protein, pea protein, rice protein, pumpkin seed protein, hemp protein, or any protein powder that you like. In many of these recipes, you can also use vanilla-flavored protein powder if you prefer.

SEEDS

- Chia seeds are another high-omega-3, high-fiber seed. They absorb their weight in liquid and can be used to create puddings and jams.

- Flaxseeds can be bought ground or whole. If you buy them whole, you'll need to grind them in a clean coffee grinder or powerful blender before using them in these recipes. They are high in plant-sourced omega-3 fatty acids and should be stored in the refrigerator or freezer until ready for use.

- Hemp seeds are the highest in protein of these seeds and can be sprinkled on oats or used in smoothies and baked goods to boost the protein content.

SPICES AND SEASONINGS

- Ground cinnamon is well known to help lower blood sugar, making it a staple for any PCOS-friendly pantry.

- Ginger is anti-inflammatory, and you can buy the root whole in the produce department or ground and dried in the spice section of your grocery store. The recipes in this book use both forms.

- Similarly, turmeric is an anti-inflammatory root that can be purchased whole in the produce department or ground and dried in the spice section. The recipes in this book use the dried and ground form.

- Tamari is a Japanese soy sauce, and gluten-free versions are available. If you prefer, feel free to substitute coconut aminos or regular soy sauce.

TEAS

- Matcha is a powdered green tea, so, unlike most teas, you do not have to brew it. Matcha can be found in many markets now as well as online.

- Spearmint tea is highly beneficial for PCOS, with studies suggesting it may help lower androgens. It is important to buy pure spearmint tea, which can be found at health food stores or online.

YOGURT

- For dairy yogurt, you want to look for plain low-sugar or no-added-sugar yogurt (such as Greek or Icelandic yogurt). Note that yogurt contains natural milk sugars (lactose). For PCOS, you want to avoid fat-free yogurt and buy full-fat varieties. Dairy products contain hormones, and the estrogen is stored in the fat, so when the fat is skimmed, all that remains is the androgens—exactly what you don't need more of with PCOS.

- When buying nondairy yogurt, read the ingredients closely. Many brands are low in protein and high in sugar, but there are better ones on the market that have around 7 grams of protein per serving.

CUSTOMIZING MEALS: INGREDIENT SWAPS

If you or anyone in your family has special dietary needs, you can easily customize the recipes in this book using the tips in this section.

DAIRY-FREE SWAPS

- All the recipes in this book that include milk call for nondairy milk. In most cases, you can use any unsweetened dairy-free milk that you like—almond, coconut, soy, pea, cashew, etc. If I feel that a certain type works best in a particular recipe, then the ingredient list will suggest a specific type.

- If a recipe calls for cheese, you can omit it completely or substitute an equal amount of store-bought or homemade dairy-free cheese.

- If a recipe calls for Greek yogurt, you can swap in plain nondairy yogurt, but note that most dairy-free yogurts are very low in protein, so using one in place of Greek yogurt will reduce the amount of protein in the recipe.

GLUTEN-FREE SWAPS

- If a recipe calls for a gluten-containing grain (such as barley), you can substitute an equal amount of brown rice or quinoa.

PROTEIN SWAPS

- If a recipe calls for a ground or whole meat that you do not have or do not want to use, you can substitute an equal amount of the ground or whole protein of your choice. For example, if you don't eat chicken, you can substitute an equal amount of tofu.

- If a recipe calls for a fish or seafood that you do not have access to or do not like, you can substitute an equal amount of the protein of your choice (although you will miss out on the anti-inflammatory benefits of the omega-3s).

FAT SWAPS

- If a recipe calls for an oil that you do not have, feel free to swap in an alternative oil or cooking fat. For example, you can swap olive oil for avocado oil or use ghee or butter if you prefer. The best oils and fats for cooking are olive oil, avocado oil, coconut oil, butter, and ghee.

- If a recipe calls for a nut or nut butter that you do not have, you can substitute an equal amount of any other nut or nut butter.

FRUIT & VEGGIE SWAPS

- You can substitute a similar type of vegetable for any vegetable you do not like or do not want to use. For example, if you don't like chard, you can substitute another leafy green, like spinach or kale. Be aware that making substitutions may affect the cooking time and flavor of the dish. You may also swap in certain frozen vegetables (such as broccoli and cauliflower) for fresh.

- If a recipe calls for a fruit that you do not have or do not want to use, you can substitute any other fruit. You may also substitute frozen fruit (such as berries) for fresh.

CUSTOMIZING CARBOHYDRATE AMOUNTS

The recipes in this book were designed for a moderate carbohydrate intake, which is what I recommend for my clients with PCOS (see page 15). Depending on several factors, they may not provide enough carbs for you.

You will want to increase your carbohydrates if

- You have lean PCOS or are at or near your ideal body weight.

- You have a high activity level and work out for at least an hour a day more than two or three times a week.

- You are cooking for a partner or family member who does not have PCOS.

- You have no signs of insulin resistance.

- You find you are getting hungry less than three hours after eating a meal.

If you need to increase your carbohydrates, simply double the amount of carbs that you cook for the week. For example, in Week 1, you would double the amount of quinoa and oats, as noted. You'll find suggestions at the beginning of each week.

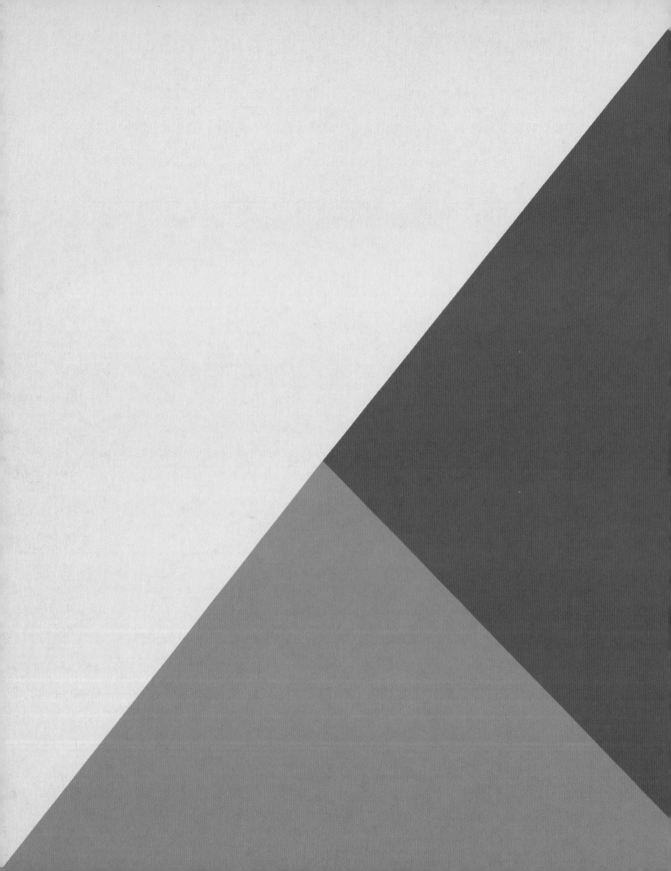

Part 1:

WEEKLY MEALS

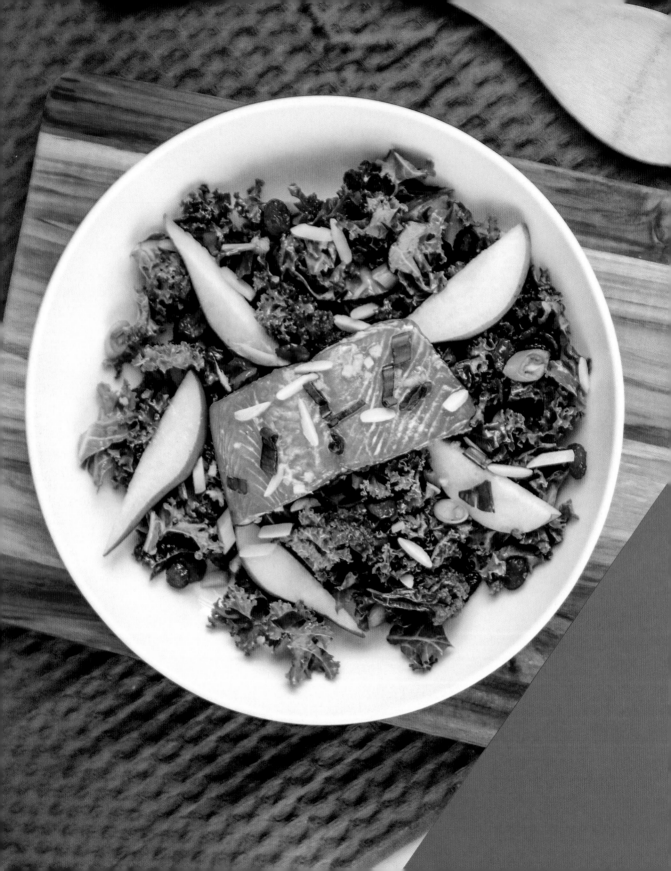

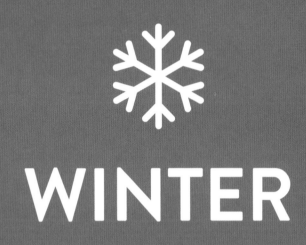

WINTER

Week 1:

SALMON, AVOCADO OIL, KALE, AND GINGER

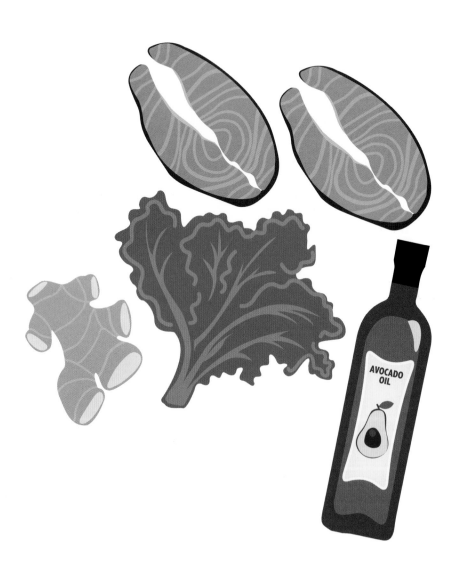

MENU

BREAKFAST	1	Gingerbread Protein Oats
	2	Mushroom, Kale, and Goat Cheese Egg Muffins
LUNCH	1	Winter Salmon Salad with Honey-Ginger Vinaigrette
	2	Asian-Inspired Kale Salad with Ginger Salmon Cakes
DINNER	1	Maple-Dijon Flax Salmon with Gingered Kale and Quinoa
	2	Ginger Salmon Cakes with Sesame Kale and Quinoa

FEATURED INGREDIENTS

 PROTEIN

This week's protein is salmon, which is especially beneficial for PCOS due to its high omega-3 fatty acid content. Omega-3 fatty acids are anti-inflammatory, and eating seafood at least twice per week has been linked to health benefits. Ideally, you want to select wild-caught salmon, as it is higher in omega-3s than farm-raised salmon. If you can't find fresh salmon locally, frozen is fine; just remember to thaw it in the refrigerator before use.

 FIBER

Curly kale is this week's fiber, and it is extremely versatile. It can be sautéed, roasted, massaged into a salad, or blended into a smoothie. Dark, leafy greens are some of the most beneficial foods you can eat with PCOS—they're full of nutrients and fiber! And unlike most leafy greens, kale is actually at its peak in the winter, after the first frost. To save time, you can buy bagged kale instead of bunches of kale.

 FAT

This week's fat is avocado oil, which is a neutral-tasting oil with a high smoke point (meaning you can cook with it at high temperatures). You can substitute it for any cooking or salad oil in any recipe where you don't want the stronger taste of olive oil or coconut oil.

 PCOS POWER FOOD

This week's PCOS Power Food is ginger, which is a potent anti-inflammatory food that adds a distinctive seasonal flavor to any recipe. If you've been intimidated by buying fresh ginger, there's no need to be! A tiny amount goes a long way. If you can't find fresh ginger near you, you can substitute ginger powder in any of the recipes.

WEEKLY INGREDIENTS

FRESH PRODUCE

Button mushrooms, whole or sliced, 8 ounces

Carrot, 1

Cilantro, 1 bunch

Cucumber, 1

Garlic, 5 cloves

Ginger, 1 (5-inch) piece

Green onions, 6

Kale, 2 bunches or 1 (16-ounce) bag

Pear (any type), 1

Radishes, 4

Red onions, 2

Yellow onion, 1

FROZEN FOODS

Edamame, shelled, 1 cup

MEAT/SEAFOOD

Salmon, 4 (4-ounce) fillets

EGGS/DAIRY/MILK

Eggs, 10 large

Goat cheese, 2 ounces

Unsweetened nondairy milk of choice, 1½ cups plus 2 tablespoons

PANTRY

Avocado oil, ¾ cup

Blackstrap molasses, 2 teaspoons

Cooking spray (avocado or olive oil)

Dijon mustard, 1 tablespoon

Dried cranberries, ¼ cup

Ground flaxseed, ¼ cup

Honey, 1 tablespoon

Lemon juice, 2 tablespoons

Lime juice, 1 tablespoon

Maple syrup, 1 tablespoon

Old-fashioned oats, ¾ cup

Protein powder, unflavored, or collagen peptides, ¼ cup (2 scoops)

Quinoa, 1 cup

Salmon, wild pink, 2 (14.75-ounce) cans

Sesame oil, dark (toasted), 2 teaspoons

Sesame seeds, 2 tablespoons

Slivered almonds, 2 tablespoons

Tamari, 1 tablespoon plus 2 teaspoons

Vanilla extract, 1 teaspoon

Walnuts, raw, 2 tablespoons

SEASONINGS

Ground cinnamon, ½ teaspoon

Ground cloves, ¼ teaspoon

CUSTOMIZING THE PLAN

TO ADD MORE CARBS:

- Double the quinoa.
- Double the oats.

TO MAKE THIS WEEK DAIRY-FREE:

- Omit the goat cheese.

PREP DAY

Today you will be cooking the quinoa, baking some of the salmon, and prepping some of the vegetables for the week. Start with the quinoa and salmon since those take the longest to cook. Also bake the Mushroom, Kale, and Goat Cheese Egg Muffins (page 36) and precook the Gingerbread Protein Oats (page 35) so that all you have to do in the mornings is heat them up.

Note: You will need to make the Ginger Salmon Cakes with Sesame Kale and Quinoa dinner before making the Asian-Inspired Kale Salad with Ginger Salmon Cakes lunch.

Complete the following tasks and store each component in a separate container in the refrigerator for use later in the week.

COOK THE QUINOA

YIELD: about 2 cups
PREP TIME: 2 minutes
COOK TIME: about 20 minutes

Cook 1 cup quinoa according to the package instructions.

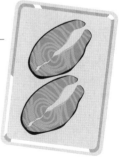

BAKE SOME OF THE SALMON

PREP TIME: 2 minutes
COOK TIME: 20 minutes

Preheat the oven to 375°F. Line a sheet pan with parchment paper or spray it with cooking spray. Place two 4-ounce salmon fillets on the prepared pan and season with salt and pepper. Bake for 20 minutes, or until the salmon is opaque in the center.

SLICE AND DICE THE YELLOW AND RED ONIONS

Dice enough yellow onion to measure ½ cup. Thinly slice enough red onion to measure 1 cup.

SLICE THE GREEN ONIONS

Thinly slice 6 green onions.

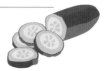

SLICE THE CARROT

Slice a carrot on the diagonal into coins.

SLICE THE CUCUMBER

Slice enough cucumber to measure ½ cup.

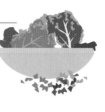

SLICE THE MUSHROOMS

Thinly slice enough button mushrooms to measure 2 cups. (If you bought presliced mushrooms, skip this step.)

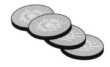

CHOP THE KALE

Roughly chop 2 bunches of kale, removing any tough stems. (If you bought prechopped kale, skip this step.)

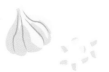

SLICE THE RADISHES

Thinly slice 4 radishes.

MINCE THE GARLIC

Mince 5 cloves of garlic.

MINCE THE GINGER

Peel and mince enough ginger to measure about ¼ cup.

CHOP THE CILANTRO

Finely chop enough cilantro to measure ½ cup. You may not need the whole bunch.

Gingerbread
PROTEIN OATS

YIELD: 2 servings
PREP TIME: 3 minutes
COOK TIME: 5 minutes

1. Put the oats, milk, and ginger in a small saucepan over medium heat and cook, stirring frequently, until the milk is absorbed, about 5 minutes.

2. Remove from the heat and stir in the protein powder, flaxseed, molasses, vanilla, cinnamon, and cloves.

3. Serve topped with the walnuts and fruit, if desired, or store for later in the week.

¾ **cup old-fashioned oats**

1½ **cups unsweetened nondairy milk of choice**

1 teaspoon minced ginger √

¼ **cup (2 scoops) unflavored protein powder**

2 tablespoons ground flaxseed

2 teaspoons molasses

1 teaspoon vanilla extract

½ **teaspoon ground cinnamon**

¼ **teaspoon ground cloves**

2 tablespoons chopped raw walnuts, for topping

Sliced apples or other fruit of choice, for topping (optional)

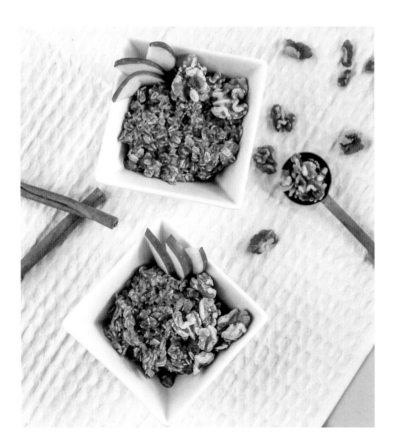

2
BREAKFAST

Mushroom, Kale, and Goat Cheese
EGG MUFFINS

YIELD: 8 muffins (2 per serving)
PREP TIME: 5 minutes
COOK TIME: 30 minutes

1 tablespoon avocado oil

½ cup diced yellow onions √

1 cup thinly sliced button mushrooms √

1 cup chopped kale √

1 clove garlic, minced √

8 large eggs

2 tablespoons unsweetened nondairy milk of choice

¼ teaspoon fine sea salt

2 ounces goat cheese

1. Preheat the oven to 350°F. Spray 8 wells of a standard-size muffin tin with cooking spray.

2. Heat the oil in a large skillet over medium-high heat. Once hot, add the onions and sauté for 3 minutes, until softened.

3. Add the mushrooms and cook until slightly browned, about 5 minutes.

4. Add the kale and garlic and cook, stirring, until the kale is wilted, about 2 minutes.

5. In a medium bowl, whisk the eggs with the milk and salt.

6. Distribute the kale and mushroom mixture evenly among the greased wells of the muffin tin. Pour the egg mixture evenly over the vegetables.

7. Crumble the goat cheese and sprinkle it over the egg mixture.

8. Bake for 20 minutes, or until firm in the center. Remove from the oven and let cool in the pan. Serve, or store in the refrigerator for later in the week.

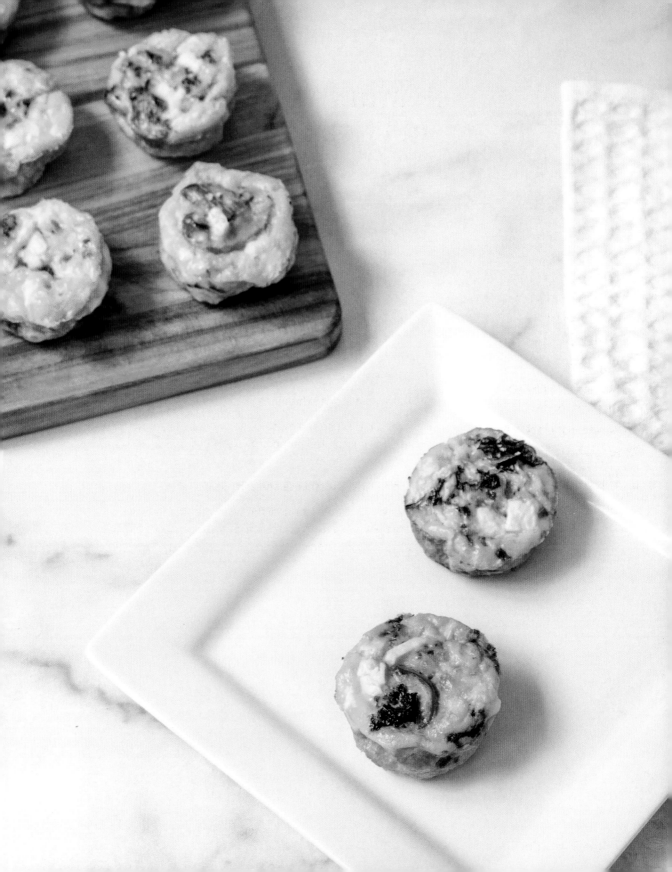

Winter Salmon Salad
with HONEY-GINGER VINAIGRETTE

YIELD: 2 servings
PREP TIME: 5 minutes
COOK TIME: —

3 cups chopped kale √

4 tablespoons avocado oil, divided

⅜ teaspoon fine sea salt, divided

1 pear (any type)

2 tablespoons lemon juice

1 tablespoon honey

1 teaspoon minced ginger √

Ground black pepper

2 (4-ounce) salmon fillets, baked √

¼ cup dried cranberries

2 tablespoons slivered almonds

2 green onions, thinly sliced √

1. Put the kale, 1 tablespoon of the oil, and ⅛ teaspoon of the salt in a large bowl. Massage with your hands until the kale has softened.

2. Core the pear and thinly slice it lengthwise; set aside.

3. Make the dressing: In a small jar, combine the remaining 3 tablespoons of oil, the lemon juice, honey, ginger, and the remaining ¼ teaspoon of salt. Season with pepper to taste.

4. Divide the kale between two plates and top each with a salmon fillet and half of the pear slices, cranberries, almonds, and green onions. Drizzle the dressing over the salads.

5. Serve, or store in the refrigerator for later in the week.

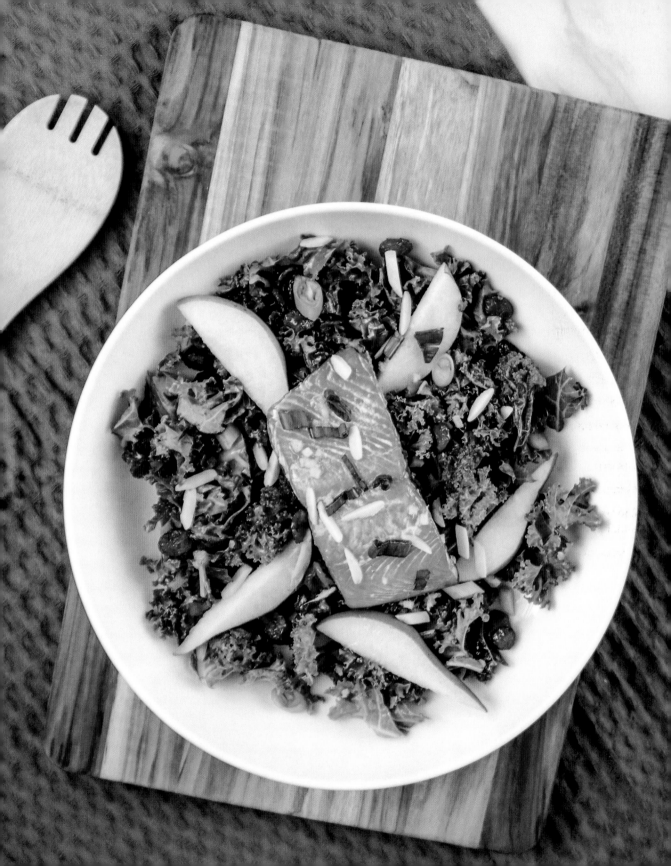

Asian-Inspired Kale Salad with
GINGER SALMON CAKES

YIELD: 2 servings
PREP TIME: 5 minutes
COOK TIME: —

1 cup frozen edamame

3 cups chopped kale √

3 tablespoons avocado oil, divided

⅛ teaspoon fine sea salt

1 tablespoon lime juice

2 teaspoons tamari

1 teaspoon dark (toasted) sesame oil

4 Ginger Salmon Cakes (page 44) √

4 radishes, thinly sliced √

½ cup cucumber slices √

2 green onions, thinly sliced √

1 tablespoon sesame seeds

1. Defrost the edamame under running water and set aside.

2. Put the kale, 1 tablespoon of the avocado oil, and the salt in a large bowl. Massage with your hands until the kale has softened.

3. Make the dressing: In a small jar, combine the remaining 2 tablespoons of avocado oil, the lime juice, tamari, and sesame oil.

4. Divide the kale between two plates and top each with two salmon cakes and half of the edamame, radishes, cucumbers, green onions, and sesame seeds. Drizzle the dressing over the salads.

5. Serve, or store in the refrigerator for later in the week.

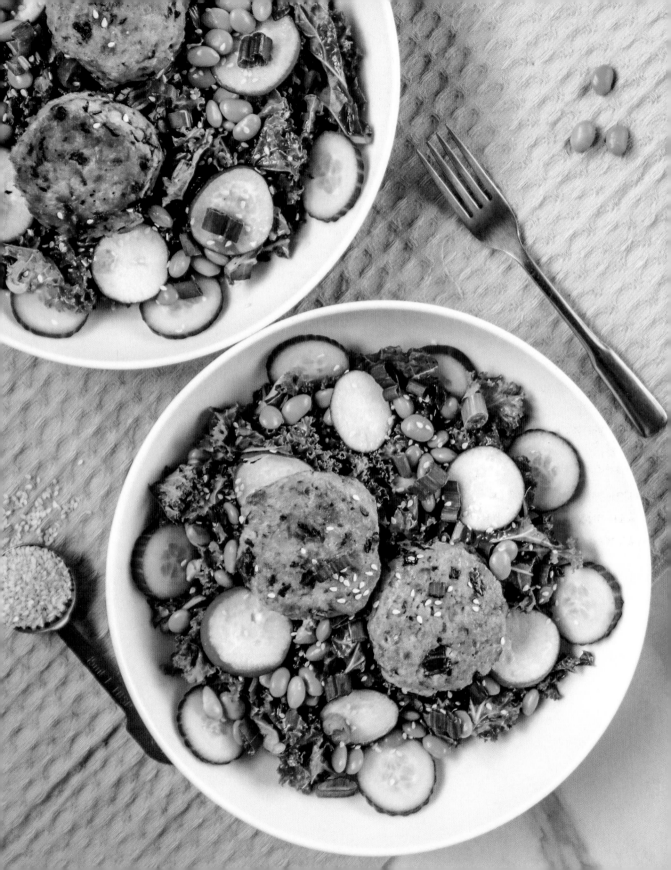

Maple-Dijon Flax Salmon
with GINGERED KALE and QUINOA

YIELD: 2 servings
PREP TIME: 5 minutes
COOK TIME: about 20 minutes

2 (4-ounce) salmon fillets

1 tablespoon Dijon mustard

1 tablespoon maple syrup

2 tablespoons ground flaxseed

2 tablespoons avocado oil, divided

½ cup diced yellow onions √

1 carrot, sliced into coins √

1 cup thinly sliced button mushrooms √

1 tablespoon minced ginger √

2 cloves garlic, minced √

2 cups chopped kale √

1 cup cooked quinoa √

1. Preheat the oven to 375°F and line a sheet pan with parchment paper.

2. Place the salmon fillets on the lined sheet pan.

3. In a small bowl, combine the mustard, maple syrup, flaxseed, and 1 tablespoon of the oil. Spread the mustard mixture on the fish.

4. Bake for 18 minutes, or until the salmon is opaque in the center.

5. Meanwhile, in a large skillet, sauté the onions in the remaining tablespoon of oil until soft, about 5 minutes.

6. Add the carrot, mushrooms, ginger, and garlic to the skillet and cook, stirring often, until the mushrooms have softened, about 3 minutes.

7. Add the kale and quinoa and cook, stirring often, until the kale has wilted and the quinoa is warmed through, about 3 minutes.

8. Divide the vegetable and quinoa mixture between two plates and top each with a salmon fillet, or store the components separately for later in the week.

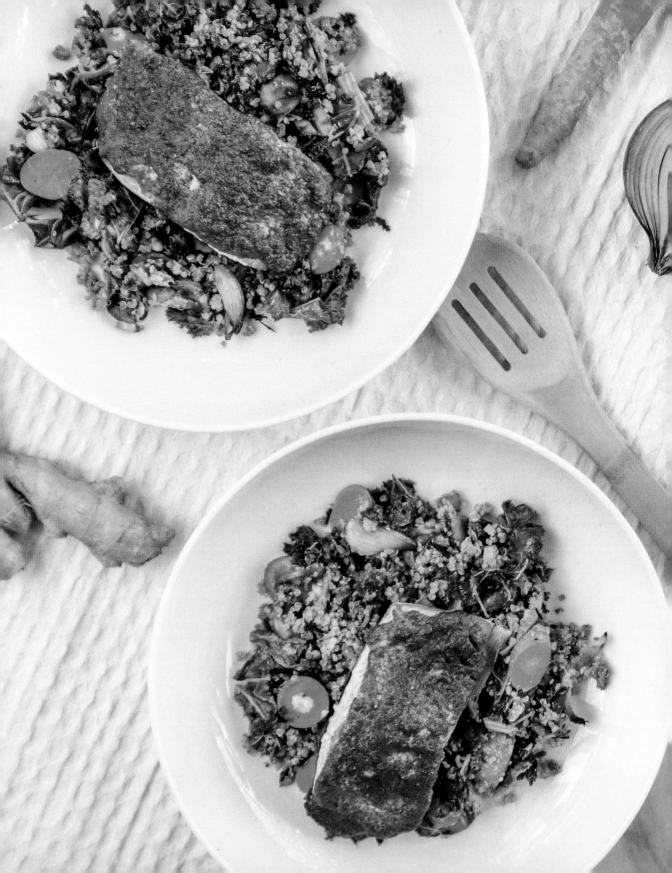

Ginger Salmon Cakes
with SESAME KALE and QUINOA

YIELD: 2 servings + 4 leftover salmon cakes
PREP TIME: 5 minutes
COOK TIME: about 20 minutes

2 (14.75-ounce) cans wild pink salmon

2 large eggs

2 green onions, thinly sliced √

½ cup chopped fresh cilantro √

2 tablespoons minced ginger √

2 tablespoons avocado oil, divided

2 cups chopped kale √

2 cloves garlic, minced √

1 tablespoon sesame seeds

1 tablespoon tamari

1 teaspoon dark (toasted) sesame oil

1 cup cooked quinoa √

1. In a large bowl, combine the salmon, eggs, green onions, cilantro, and ginger. Shape the mixture into 8 cakes, about 2 inches in diameter and 1 inch thick.

2. Heat 1 tablespoon of the avocado oil in a large skillet. When the oil is hot, carefully add the salmon cakes. Cook until lightly browned on one side, about 4 minutes, then flip carefully and cook until lightly browned on the other side.

3. Meanwhile, in another large skillet, sauté the kale in the remaining 1 tablespoon of avocado oil until soft, about 2 minutes.

4. Add the garlic, sesame seeds, tamari, and sesame oil to the skillet and stir until the garlic is fragrant, about 2 minutes.

5. Add the quinoa to the skillet with the kale mixture and cook until warmed through, about 3 minutes.

6. Store four of the salmon cakes in the refrigerator for use in the Asian-Inspired Kale Salad (page 40). Divide the kale and quinoa mixture between two plates and top each plate with two of the remaining salmon cakes, or store the components separately for later in the week.

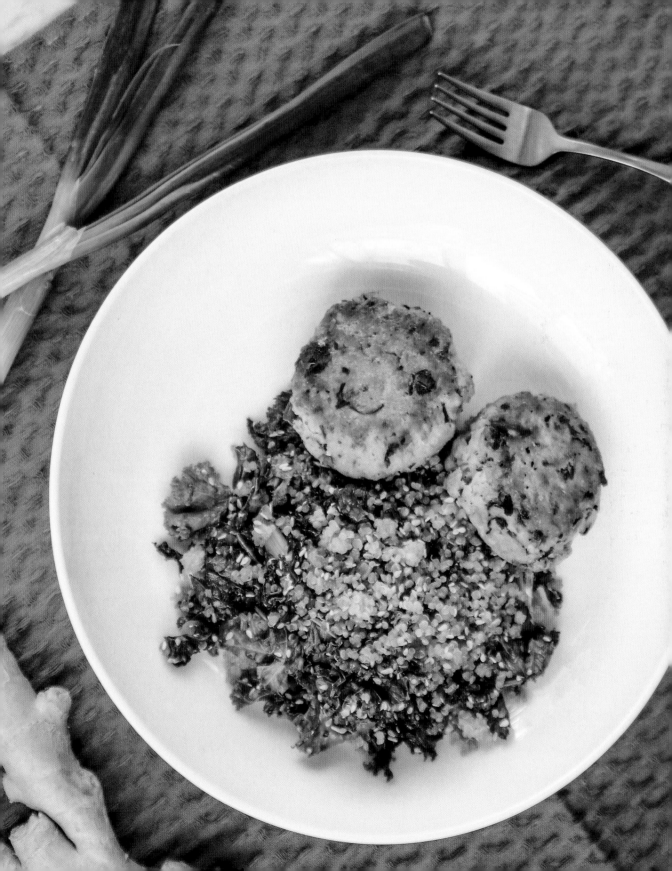

Week 2:

TURKEY CUTLETS, OLIVE OIL, PEARS, AND SWISS CHARD

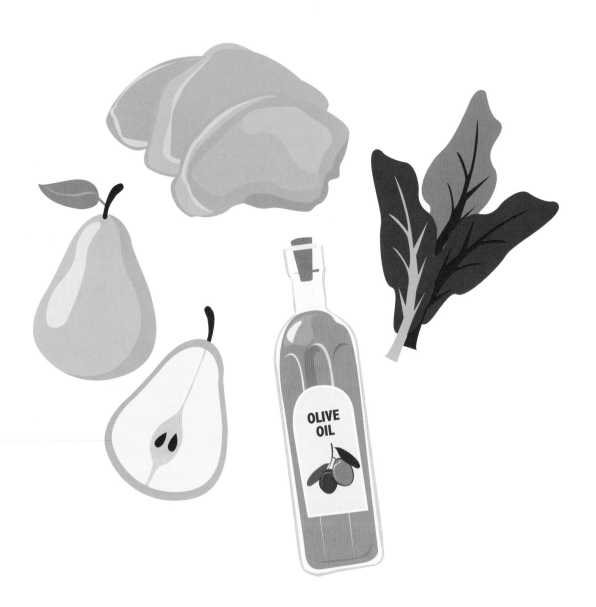

MENU

BREAKFAST	1	Pear Breakfast Crumble
	2	Cranberry Pear Protein Oats
LUNCH	1	Egg Salad–Stuffed Chard Wraps
	2	Thanksgiving Turkey Wraps
DINNER	1	Turkey Cutlets with Pear Slaw and Sautéed Chard
	2	Herbed Turkey Fingers with Sweet Potato Fries

FEATURED INGREDIENTS

PROTEIN

This week's protein is turkey cutlets, which are a versatile and affordable lean protein source. Turkey cutlets are thinly sliced turkey breast, which you can find packaged or request from your butcher. Feel free to use turkey breasts or turkey tenderloins instead.

FIBER

Pears are this week's source of fiber because they're a fiber powerhouse! One medium-sized pear contains 6 grams of fiber with only 27 grams of total carbs, making it a smart fruit choice for PCOS. There are a variety of pears available—Anjou, Bartlett, Bosc, and the less common Seckel and Comice. Use whichever pears are available locally.

FAT

This week's fat is olive oil, which is a staple of the anti-inflammatory Mediterranean diet. Extra-virgin olive oil is not only safe to cook with but also adds a delicious flavor to almost any dish.

PCOS POWER FOOD

This week's PCOS Power Food is Swiss chard, which is a dark, leafy green vegetable common in Mediterranean cooking. It comes in a variety of colors and provides a variety of nutrients important for PCOS, including high levels of magnesium and potassium. Its broad leaves are sturdy enough to be used as low-carb wraps.

WEEKLY INGREDIENTS

FRESH PRODUCE

Avocados, Hass, 2

Button mushrooms, whole or sliced, 8 ounces

Garlic, 4 cloves

Green onions, 8

Pears (any type), 6

Sweet potatoes, 2 medium

Swiss chard, 3 bunches

Yellow onions, 2 small

MEAT/SEAFOOD

Turkey cutlets, 6 (4 ounces each)

EGGS/DAIRY/MILK

Eggs, 8 large

Greek yogurt, full-fat plain, 2 cups (optional, for Pear Breakfast Crumble)

Unsweetened nondairy milk of choice, 1½ cups

PANTRY

Almond meal, ¾ cup plus 2 tablespoons

Apple cider vinegar, 2 tablespoons

Coconut oil, ¼ cup

Collagen peptides or unflavored protein powder, ½ cup (4 scoops)

Cooking spray (avocado or olive oil)

Dijon mustard, ¼ cup

Dried cranberries, ½ cup

Ground flaxseed, ½ cup

Hemp seeds, hulled, ¼ cup plus 2 tablespoons

Lemon juice, 3 tablespoons

Maple syrup, 2 tablespoons

Old-fashioned oats, ¾ cup

Olive oil, extra-virgin, ¼ cup plus 2 tablespoons

Vanilla extract, 1 teaspoon

SEASONINGS

Dried parsley, 1 teaspoon

Ginger powder, 1 teaspoon

Ground cinnamon, 1½ teaspoons

Italian seasoning, 2 teaspoons

CUSTOMIZING THE PLAN

TO ADD MORE CARBS:

- Double the oats.
- Double the sweet potatoes.
- Use whole-grain wraps in place of the Swiss chard leaves in the two wraps.

TO MAKE THIS WEEK DAIRY-FREE:

- Use a nondairy yogurt in place of the Greek yogurt.

PREP DAY

Today you will be baking the sweet potato fries and some of the turkey, boiling the eggs, and prepping some of the vegetables for the week. Start with the sweet potato fries and turkey since you can prep the rest of the vegetables while they cook. Also bake the Pear Breakfast Crumble (page 51) and precook the Cranberry Pear Protein Oats (page 52) so that all you have to do in the mornings is heat them up.

Complete the following tasks and store each component in a separate container in the refrigerator for use later in the week.

BAKE THE SWEET POTATO FRIES

YIELD: about 2 cups
PREP TIME: 2 minutes
COOK TIME: 30 minutes

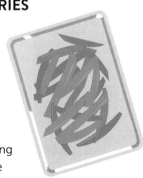

Preheat the oven to 375°F. Peel and slice 2 medium sweet potatoes lengthwise into 4 by ½ by ½-inch sticks. Spray a sheet pan with cooking spray and place the potatoes on the pan. Season with salt and pepper. Bake, turning halfway through, until slightly browned, about 30 minutes.

BAKE SOME OF THE TURKEY

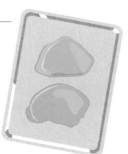

PREP TIME: 2 minutes
COOK TIME: 25 minutes

Spray a sheet pan with cooking spray and place two 4-ounce turkey cutlets on it. Season the turkey with salt and pepper. Put the pan in the oven next to the sweet potatoes and bake for 25 minutes, or until cooked through.

HARD-BOIL SOME OF THE EGGS

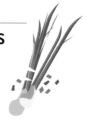

PREP TIME: 2 minutes
COOK TIME: 10 minutes

Put 6 eggs in a medium saucepan and cover completely with water. Bring to a boil over medium-high heat. When the water reaches a boil, turn off the heat and let the eggs sit in the hot water for 10 minutes. Drain the hot water and fill the pan with cold water. When the eggs are cool, peel them.

SLICE THE YELLOW ONION

Slice enough yellow onion to measure 1 cup.

SLICE THE GREEN ONIONS

Thinly slice 8 green onions.

SLICE THE MUSHROOMS

Thinly slice enough button mushrooms to measure 2 cups. (If you bought presliced mushrooms, skip this step.)

MINCE THE GARLIC

Mince 4 cloves of garlic.

Pear Breakfast
CRUMBLE

YIELD: 4 servings
PREP TIME: 5 minutes
COOK TIME: 30 minutes

1. Preheat the oven to 400°F. Spray an 8-inch square baking pan with cooking spray.

2. Halve, core, and thinly slice the pears; layer them in the prepared pan. Sprinkle with the lemon juice.

3. Make the topping: Put the almond meal, flaxseed, collagen, cinnamon, and ginger in a large bowl and stir to combine. Add the coconut oil, maple syrup, and vanilla and stir. The mixture should be crumbly.

4. Crumble the topping mixture over the pears. Bake for 30 minutes, or until the topping is golden brown. Remove from the oven and let cool.

5. Serve topped with the yogurt, if desired, or store in the refrigerator for later in the week.

4 pears (any type)

2 tablespoons lemon juice

½ cup almond meal

¼ cup ground flaxseed

¼ cup (2 scoops) collagen peptides or unflavored protein powder

1 teaspoon ground cinnamon

½ teaspoon ginger powder

¼ cup coconut oil, melted

2 tablespoons maple syrup

1 teaspoon vanilla extract

2 cups full-fat plain Greek yogurt, for serving (optional)

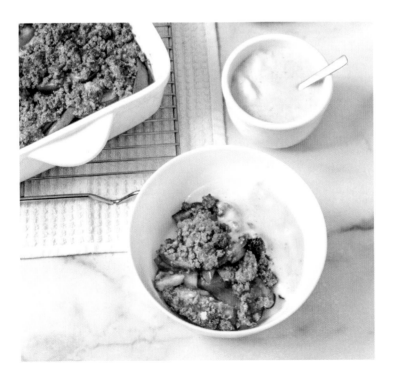

Cranberry Pear
PROTEIN OATS

YIELD: 2 servings
PREP TIME: 3 minutes
COOK TIME: 8 minutes

¾ cup old-fashioned oats

1½ cups unsweetened nondairy milk of choice

1 pear (any type)

¼ cup (2 scoops) collagen peptides or unflavored protein powder

¼ cup dried cranberries

2 tablespoons almond meal

2 tablespoons hulled hemp seeds

½ teaspoon ground cinnamon

½ teaspoon ginger powder

1. Put the oats and milk in a small saucepan over medium heat and cook, stirring frequently, until the milk is absorbed, about 5 minutes.

2. Finely dice the pear and add it to the pan with the oats. Stir and cook until the pear is warmed through, about 3 minutes.

3. Remove from the heat and stir in the collagen, cranberries, almond meal, hemp seeds, cinnamon, and ginger.

4. Serve, or store in the refrigerator for later in the week.

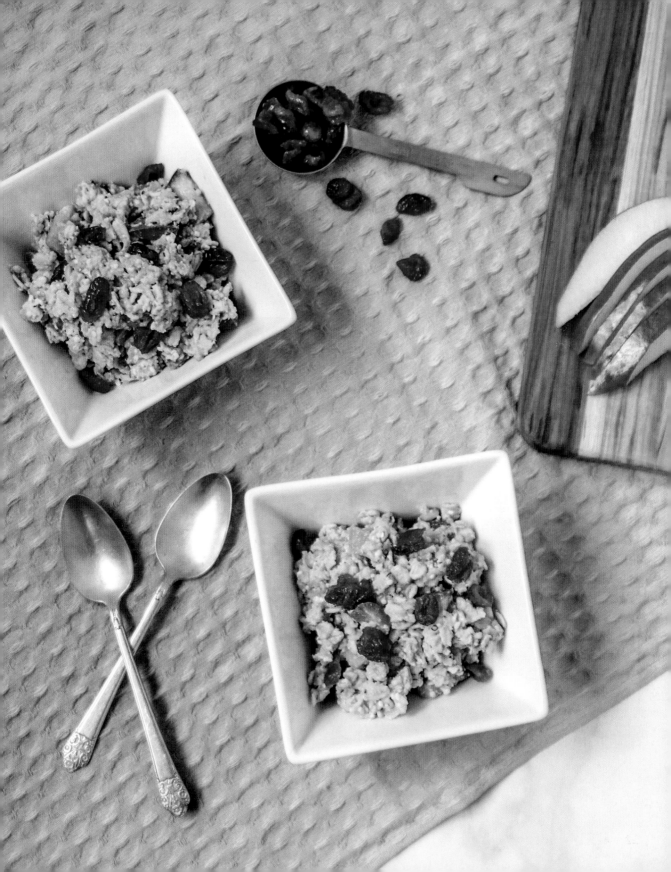

YIELD: 2 servings
PREP TIME: 10 minutes
COOK TIME: —

Egg Salad–Stuffed
CHARD WRAPS

1 Hass avocado

2 tablespoons Dijon mustard

1 tablespoon extra-virgin olive oil

2 teaspoons lemon juice

6 hard-boiled eggs, peeled √

4 green onions, thinly sliced √

Salt and pepper

4 large Swiss chard leaves

1. Halve the avocado, remove the pit, and scoop the flesh into a large bowl. Add the mustard, oil, and lemon juice and mash until smooth.

2. Roughly chop the eggs. Add the eggs and green onions to the bowl with the avocado mixture and stir well. Season with salt and pepper to taste.

3. To serve, remove the stems from the chard leaves and place two leaves on each of two plates. Fill each leaf with one-quarter of the egg salad and wrap the leaves tightly around the filling.

4. Serve, or store in the refrigerator for later in the week.

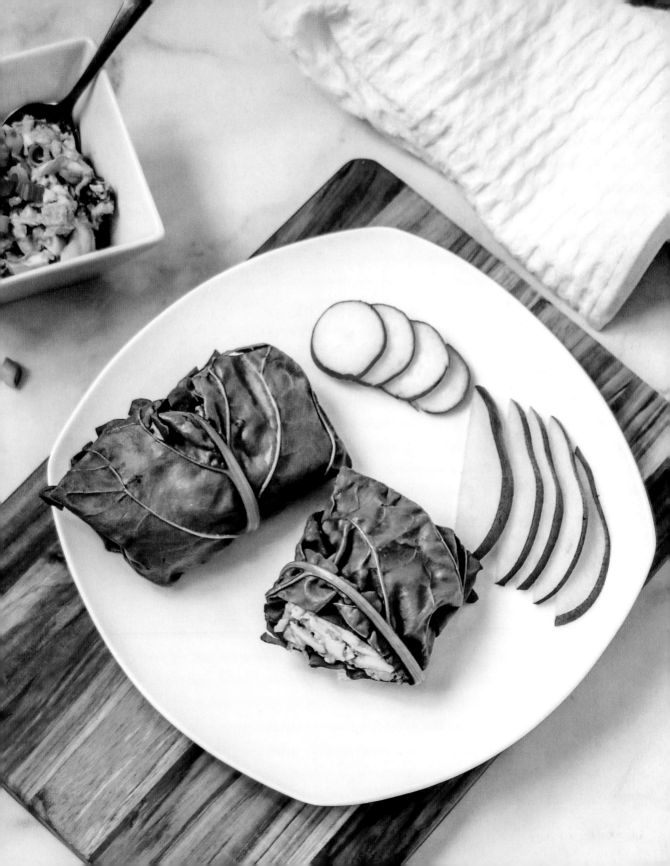

Thanksgiving
TURKEY WRAPS

YIELD: 2 servings

PREP TIME: 5 minutes

COOK TIME: —

1 Hass avocado

2 tablespoons Dijon mustard

1 tablespoon extra-virgin olive oil

1 teaspoon lemon juice

Salt and pepper

2 (4-ounce) turkey cutlets, baked √

2 large Swiss chard leaves

1 cup sweet potato fries √

¼ cup dried cranberries

1. Halve the avocado, remove the pit, and scoop the flesh into a medium bowl. Add the mustard, oil, and lemon juice and mash until smooth. Season with salt and pepper to taste.

2. Slice the turkey cutlets into ¾-inch strips.

3. Remove the stems from the chard leaves and place a leaf on each of two plates. Layer each leaf with half of the avocado mixture, turkey, sweet potato fries, and cranberries. Wrap the leaves tightly around the filling.

4. Serve, or store in the refrigerator for later in the week.

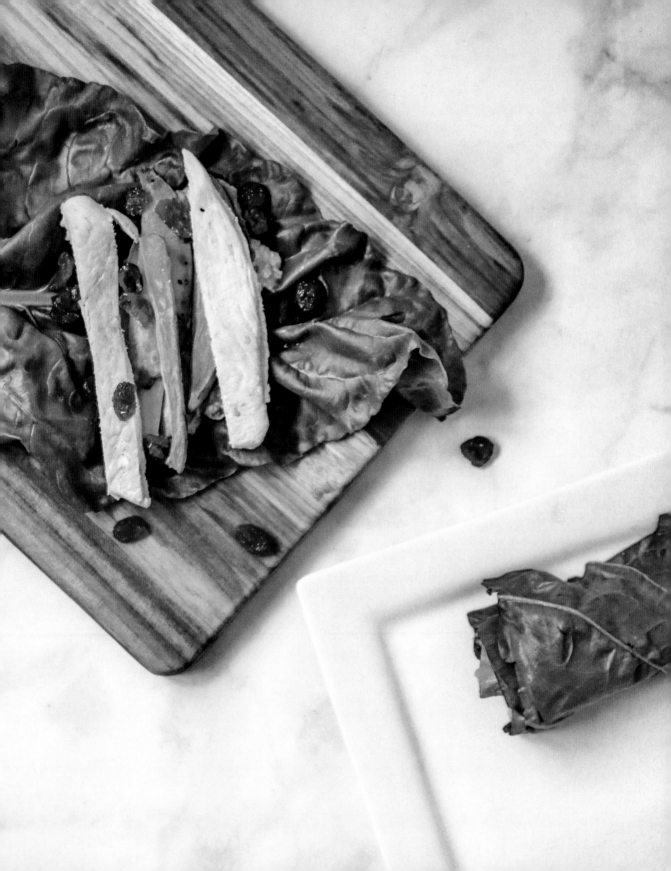

Turkey Cutlets with
PEAR SLAW and
SAUTÉED CHARD

YIELD: 2 servings + about 2 cups leftover sautéed chard
PREP TIME: 5 minutes
COOK TIME: about 25 minutes

1 cup sliced yellow onions √

3 tablespoons extra-virgin olive oil, divided

2 bunches Swiss chard

2 (4-ounce) turkey cutlets

2 cups thinly sliced button mushrooms √

4 cloves garlic, minced √

4 green onions, thinly sliced √

1 teaspoon dried parsley

Fine sea salt

Ground black pepper

2 tablespoons apple cider vinegar, divided

1 pear (any type)

1. Make the sautéed chard: In a large sauté pan over medium heat, sauté the onions in 1 tablespoon of the oil until golden brown, about 5 minutes.

2. Roughly chop the chard. Add the stems to the pan with the onions and cook for about 5 minutes, until softened. Add the green tops and cook, stirring, until wilted. Remove the pan from the heat and set aside.

3. Meanwhile, in a medium skillet, heat 1 tablespoon of the oil until hot. Add the turkey cutlets and cook for 5 to 6 minutes on each side, until slightly browned and cooked through. Remove from the pan and set aside.

4. In the same skillet, cook the mushrooms until softened, about 5 minutes. Add the garlic, green onions, and parsley and cook, stirring, until the garlic is fragrant. Season with salt and pepper to taste. Stir in 1 tablespoon of the vinegar and remove from the heat.

5. Make the slaw: Core and thinly slice the pear and put the slices in a medium bowl. Add the remaining tablespoon of vinegar and remaining tablespoon of oil and toss to coat. Season with salt and pepper to taste.

6. Store half of the sautéed chard in the refrigerator for use in the Herbed Turkey Fingers with Sweet Potato Fries (page 60). Divide the remaining greens evenly between two plates. Top with the turkey and mushroom mixture and serve the pear slaw on the side.

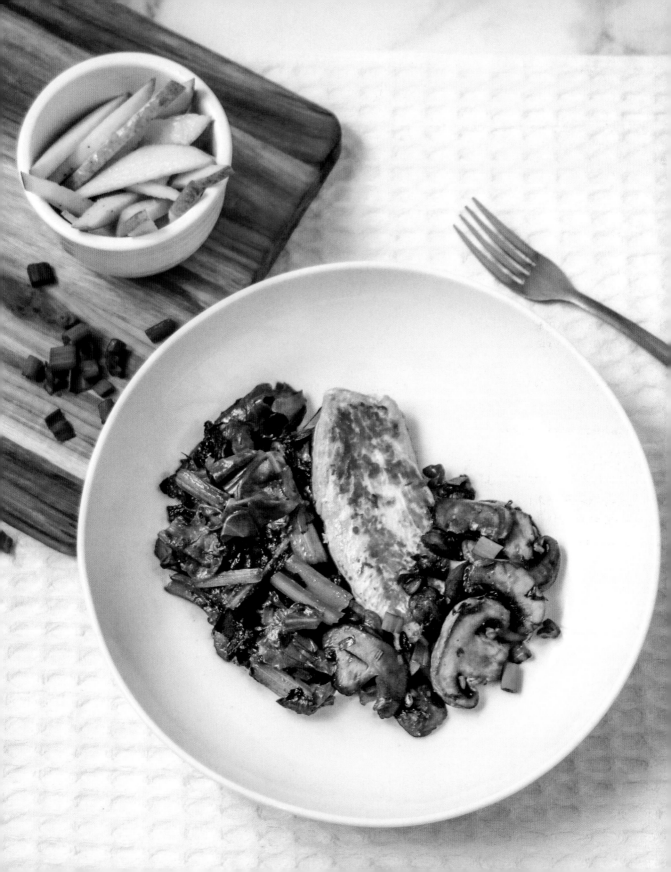

Herbed Turkey Fingers
with SWEET POTATO FRIES

YIELD: 2 servings
PREP TIME: 5 minutes
COOK TIME: about 20 minutes

2 (4-ounce) turkey cutlets

2 large eggs

¼ cup almond meal

¼ cup ground flaxseed

2 teaspoons Italian seasoning

¼ teaspoon salt

Half of the sweet potato fries (about 1 cup) √

1 tablespoon extra-virgin olive oil

2 cups sautéed Swiss chard (page 58) √

Dipping sauce of choice (such as barbecue or honey mustard), for serving

1. Preheat the oven to 400°F. Line a sheet pan with parchment paper.

2. Slice each turkey cutlet into five equal-sized strips.

3. In a small bowl, whisk the eggs. Put the almond meal, flaxseed, Italian seasoning, and salt in a separate shallow dish and stir to combine.

4. Dredge each strip of turkey in the egg, then in the almond meal mixture, and place on the prepared sheet pan.

5. Bake the turkey fingers for 30 minutes, or until cooked through and golden brown.

6. Meanwhile, on a separate sheet pan, toss the sweet potato fries with the oil. Put the pan in the oven when the turkey has 10 minutes left to cook.

7. While the turkey and fries are in the oven, heat the leftover sautéed chard in the microwave or on the stovetop.

8. Serve the turkey fingers with the fries and greens and the dipping sauce of your choice.

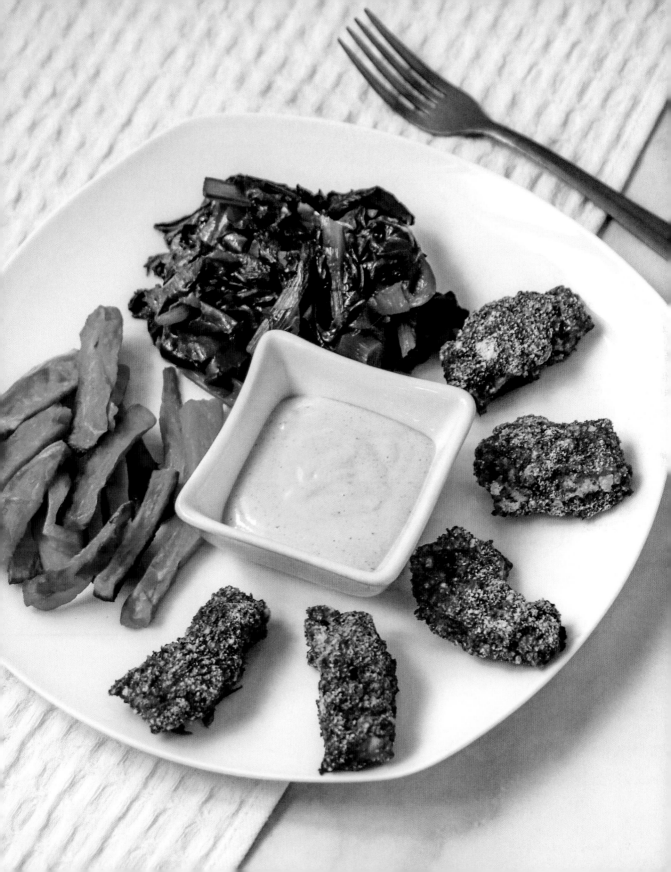

Week 3:

COD, SUNFLOWER SEEDS, RED LENTILS, AND TURNIPS

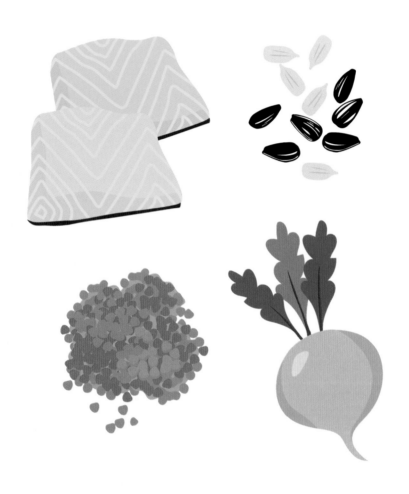

MENU

BREAKFAST	1	Sunbutter Breakfast Cookies
	2	Eggs with Root Vegetable Hash
LUNCH	1	Winter Vegetable Lentil Stew
	2	Cod Cake Lettuce Wraps
DINNER	1	Lentil Meatballs with Zucchini Noodles
	2	Cod Cakes with Roasted Root Vegetables

FEATURED INGREDIENTS

PROTEIN

This week's protein is cod, which is a lean fish that is firm and flaky when cooked. If you cannot find fresh cod locally, use any white fish instead.

FIBER

Red lentils are this week's main source of fiber. One cup of cooked lentils contains a whopping 16 grams of dietary fiber in addition to 18 grams of protein. Lentils are also a good source of many vitamins and minerals, including iron and magnesium. If you can't find red lentils, it's fine to substitute brown, green, or yellow lentils in these recipes.

FAT

This week's fat is sunflower seeds, which you'll find in the recipes both whole and in the form of sunflower seed butter. Sunflower seeds are high in many nutrients important for PCOS, including B vitamins, iron, magnesium, anti-inflammatory vitamin E, selenium, and zinc. Look for roasted unsalted whole sunflower seeds and unsweetened sunflower seed butter. (SunButter is one brand.)

PCOS POWER FOOD

This week's PCOS Power Food is turnips. This budget-friendly winter vegetable has many benefits for PCOS. Turnips are low in carbs, with only 8 grams of carbs per cup, 3 grams of which is fiber. They are also a cruciferous vegetable, related to broccoli and cauliflower, which may help your liver metabolize estrogen more efficiently. Purple-top turnips are the most common, and they are delicious roasted, sautéed, added to soups, or mashed in place of potatoes.

WEEKLY INGREDIENTS

FRESH PRODUCE

Avocado, Hass, 1

Beets, 2 medium

Carrots, 3

Garlic, 4 cloves

Green beans, 6 ounces

Green leaf lettuce, 1 head

Green onions, 4

Kale, curly, 1 bunch

Parsley, curly or Italian, 1 bunch

Radishes, 4

Red bell pepper, 1

Red cabbage, ¼ cup shredded

Sweet potato, 1 medium

Turnips, 5

Yellow onions, 6 medium

Zucchini noodles, 4 cups

MEAT/SEAFOOD

Cod or other white fish fillets, 1 pound

EGGS/DAIRY/MILK

Eggs, 7 large

PANTRY

Almond meal, ½ cup

Balsamic vinegar, 1 tablespoon

Bone broth, beef or chicken, 4 cups

Collagen peptides or unflavored protein powder, ¼ cup (2 scoops)

Cooking spray (avocado or olive oil)

Dijon mustard, 1 tablespoon plus 1 teaspoon

Ground flaxseed, 1 cup

Hemp seeds, hulled, 2 tablespoons

Maple syrup, 3 tablespoons

Old-fashioned oats, ½ cup

Olive oil, extra-virgin, ¼ cup plus 3 tablespoons

Red lentils, 1¼ cups

Sunflower seed butter, unsweetened, 1 cup

Sunflower seeds, roasted and unsalted, 2 tablespoons

Tomato paste, 2 tablespoons

Tomato sauce, 1 (15-ounce) can

Vanilla extract, 1 teaspoon

SEASONINGS

Dried basil, 1 tablespoon

Dried parsley, 2 teaspoons

Ground cinnamon, ½ teaspoon

Italian seasoning, 1 teaspoon

Turmeric powder, 1 teaspoon

CUSTOMIZING THE PLAN

TO ADD MORE CARBS:

- Double the lentils.

- Double the root vegetables (beets, sweet potatoes, and turnips).

- Use whole-grain wraps in place of the lettuce leaves in the Cod Cake Lettuce Wraps.

- Use whole-grain pasta in place of the zucchini noodles in the Lentil Meatballs.

- Add some cooked brown rice or quinoa to the Cod Cakes with Roasted Root Vegetables.

PREP DAY

Today you will be roasting the root vegetables, cooking the lentils, and prepping some of the other vegetables for the week. Start with the root vegetables and lentils and prep the remainder of the veggies while they cook. Also bake the Sunbutter Breakfast Cookies (page 67) so you have them ready for the week.

Note: You will need to make the Cod Cakes with Roasted Root Vegetables dinner before making the Cod Cake Lettuce Wraps lunch.

Complete the following tasks and store each component in a separate container in the refrigerator for use later in the week.

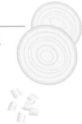

DICE THE YELLOW ONIONS

Dice enough yellow onions to measure 3½ cups. Set aside 1 cup for roasting today and store the remaining 2½ cups in the refrigerator.

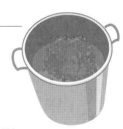

COOK THE LENTILS

YIELD: 2½ cups
PREP TIME: 2 minutes
COOK TIME: 20 minutes

Put 1¼ cups red lentils and 2½ cups water in a stockpot over medium-high heat. Bring to a boil, then lower the heat to medium and cover. The lentils are done when all of the water is absorbed, about 15 minutes. Season with salt to taste after cooking.

ROAST THE ROOT VEGETABLES

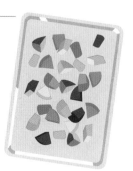

PREP TIME: 10 minutes
COOK TIME: 30 minutes

Preheat the oven to 400°F and spray a sheet pan with cooking spray. Peel and dice enough beets, sweet potatoes, and turnips to measure 1 cup each. Spread the vegetables in a single layer on the prepared pan, along with 1 cup of diced onions. Drizzle with 1 tablespoon extra-virgin olive oil and 1 tablespoon balsamic vinegar. Season with salt and pepper. Roast, stirring halfway through, until slightly browned, about 30 minutes.

CHOP THE KALE

Roughly chop enough kale to measure 2 cups, removing any tough stems.

DICE THE BELL PEPPER

Dice enough red bell pepper to measure ½ cup.

SLICE THE RADISHES

Thinly slice 4 radishes.

MINCE THE GARLIC

Mince 4 cloves of garlic.

GRATE AND DICE THE TURNIPS AND CARROTS

Use a box grater or food processor to grate enough turnips to measure 2 cups and enough carrots to measure ½ cup. Store the grated turnips and carrots together in one container. Dice enough carrots to measure 1 cup and store separately.

CHOP THE GREEN BEANS

Trim the green beans, then cut them into 1-inch pieces until you have enough to measure 1 cup.

SLICE THE GREEN ONIONS

Thinly slice 4 green onions.

CHOP THE PARSLEY

Finely chop enough fresh parsley to measure ½ cup.

PREPARE THE ZUCCHINI NOODLES

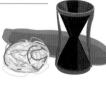

Use a spiral slicer or vegetable peeler to make 4 cups of zucchini "noodles." (If you bought prepared zucchini noodles, skip this step.)

Sunbutter
BREAKFAST COOKIES

YIELD: 8 cookies (2 per serving)
PREP TIME: 5 minutes
COOK TIME: 15 minutes

1. Preheat the oven to 350°F and line a cookie sheet with parchment paper.

2. Put all of the ingredients in a large bowl and stir until well combined.

3. Using your hands, shape the dough into 8 balls, about 1½ inches in diameter, and place on the lined cookie sheet. Gently flatten the cookies with a fork.

4. Bake for 13 to 15 minutes, until golden brown. Remove from the oven, transfer to a cooling rack, and let cool.

5. Serve, or store in the refrigerator for later in the week.

¾ cup unsweetened sunflower seed butter

2 tablespoons maple syrup

1 large egg

1 teaspoon vanilla extract

½ cup ground flaxseed

½ cup old-fashioned oats

¼ cup (2 scoops) collagen peptides or unflavored protein powder

2 tablespoons hulled hemp seeds

½ teaspoon ground cinnamon

Pinch of fine sea salt

NOTE:
These cookies freeze well, so you can freeze any leftovers that you do not plan on eating within the week.

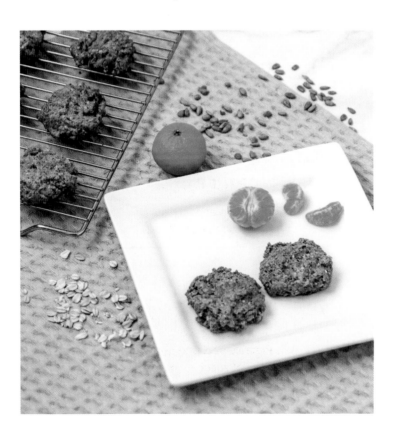

Eggs with
ROOT VEGETABLE HASH

YIELD: 2 servings
PREP TIME: 5 minutes
COOK TIME: 10 minutes

1 cup diced yellow onions √

1 tablespoon extra-virgin olive oil

2 cups chopped kale √

2 cups grated turnips √

½ cup grated carrots √

2 cloves garlic, minced √

1 teaspoon dried parsley

Salt and pepper

4 large eggs

1. Make the hash: In a large skillet, sauté the onions in the oil over medium-high heat until softened, about 3 minutes. Add the kale, turnips, carrots, garlic, and parsley, season with salt and pepper to taste, and cook until the vegetables are soft, about 3 minutes.

2. Meanwhile, spray a separate skillet with cooking spray and cook the eggs to your liking over medium-high heat.

3. Divide the hash between two plates and top each plate with two eggs.

4. Serve, or store the hash in the refrigerator for later in the week.

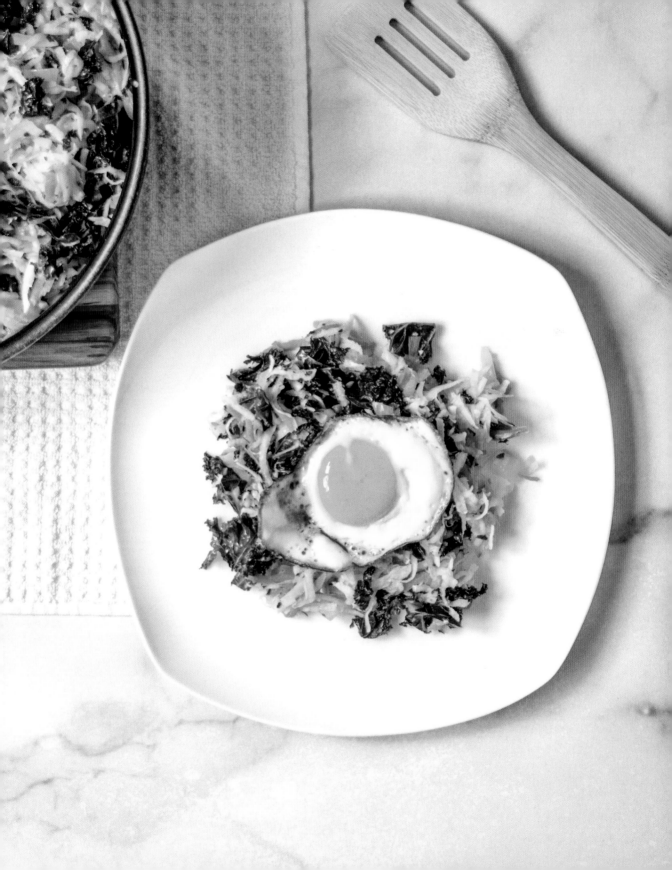

Winter Vegetable
LENTIL STEW

YIELD: 4 servings
PREP TIME: 5 minutes
COOK TIME: 25 minutes

1 cup diced yellow onions √

2 tablespoons extra-virgin olive oil, divided

2 cloves garlic, minced √

1 cup diced carrots √

1 cup diced turnips √

4 cups beef bone broth

1 teaspoon dried parsley

2 cups cooked red lentils √

1 cup chopped green beans √

1 tablespoon maple syrup

1 tablespoon Dijon mustard

1 teaspoon turmeric powder

¼ teaspoon fine sea salt

⅛ teaspoon ground black pepper

NOTE:
This stew freezes well, so you can freeze any that you don't plan on eating within the week.

1. In a stockpot, sauté the onions in 1 tablespoon of the oil over medium-high heat until softened, about 3 minutes.

2. Add the garlic and cook until fragrant, about 1 minute.

3. Add the carrots, turnips, broth, and parsley, cover, and cook until the vegetables are tender, about 15 minutes.

4. Add the lentils, green beans, maple syrup, mustard, turmeric, salt, and pepper and cook until the lentils are warmed through, about 5 minutes.

5. Serve, or store in the refrigerator for later in the week.

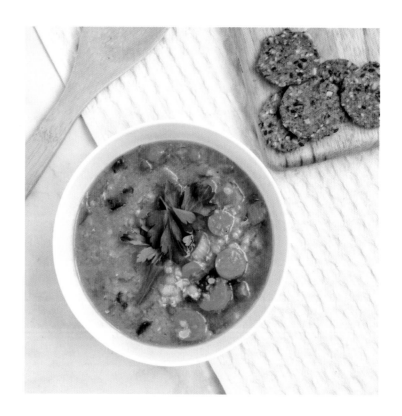

Cod Cake
LETTUCE WRAPS

YIELD: 2 servings
PREP TIME: 5 minutes
COOK TIME: —

1. Place a lettuce leaf on each of two plates.

2. Top each leaf with a cod cake and half of the radishes, cabbage, green onions, and avocado.

3. Top with the remaining lettuce leaves and eat immediately, or store in the refrigerator for later in the week.

4 leaves green lettuce

2 cod cakes (page 74)

4 radishes, thinly sliced √

¼ cup shredded red cabbage √

2 green onions, thinly sliced √

½ Hass avocado, sliced

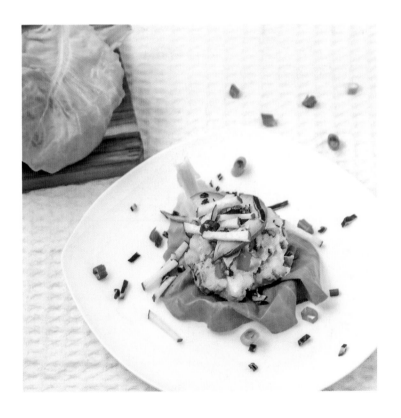

YIELD: 2 servings + 8 leftover meatballs
PREP TIME: 10 minutes
COOK TIME: 20 minutes

Lentil Meatballs with
ZUCCHINI NOODLES

1½ cups cooked red lentils √

½ cup ground flaxseed

¼ cup unsweetened sunflower seed butter

1 large egg

1 teaspoon Italian seasoning

2 tablespoons tomato paste, divided

¼ teaspoon fine sea salt, divided

½ cup diced yellow onions √

2 tablespoons extra-virgin olive oil, divided

2 cloves garlic, minced √

1 (15-ounce) can tomato sauce

1 tablespoon dried basil

4 cups zucchini noodles √

1. Preheat the oven to 375°F. Line a sheet pan with parchment paper.

2. In a large bowl, combine the lentils, flaxseed, sunflower seed butter, egg, Italian seasoning, 1 tablespoon of the tomato paste, and ⅛ teaspoon of the salt. Using wet hands, roll the mixture into sixteen 1-inch balls and place on the prepared pan. Bake for 20 minutes, or until cooked through.

3. Meanwhile, in a large skillet over medium-high heat, sauté the onions in 1 tablespoon of the oil until softened, about 3 minutes. Add the garlic and cook for 1 minute, until fragrant.

4. Add the tomato sauce, the remaining tablespoon of tomato paste, the basil, and the remaining ⅛ teaspoon salt. Reduce the heat to low and cook until the sauce is warmed through.

5. In another large skillet, heat the remaining tablespoon of oil over medium-high heat. Add the zucchini noodles and cook, tossing frequently, until softened, about 3 minutes.

6. Divide the zucchini noodles between two plates. Top each plate with four lentil meatballs and half of the sauce. Store the remaining meatballs for later in the week, or freeze for later use.

NOTE:
These meatballs freeze well, so you can freeze any that you don't plan on eating within the week.

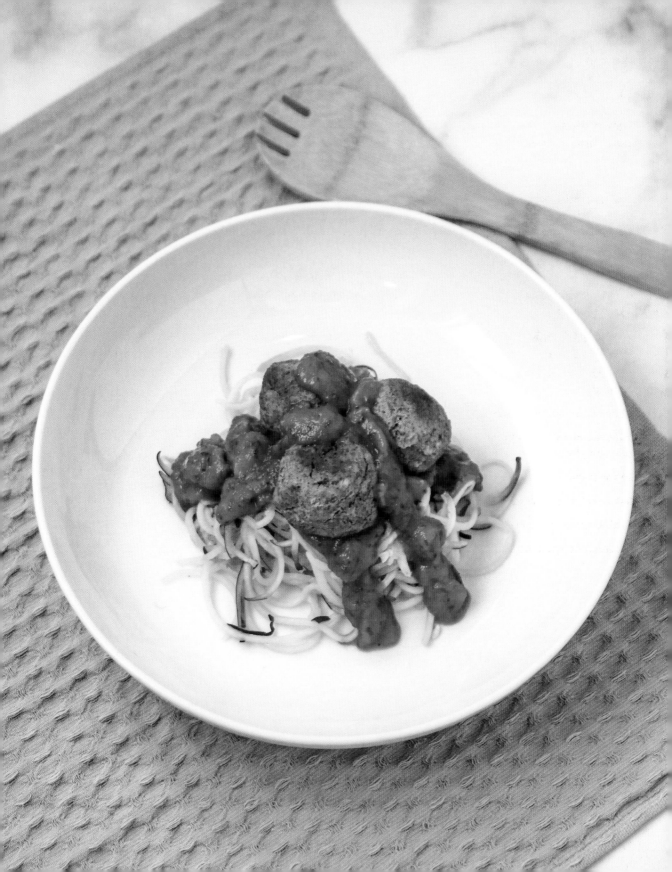

Cod Cakes with
ROASTED ROOT VEGETABLES

YIELD: 2 servings + 2 leftover cod cakes
PREP TIME: 5 minutes
COOK TIME: 25 minutes

1 pound cod or other white fish fillets

1 large egg

½ cup almond meal

½ cup diced red bell peppers √

2 green onions, thinly sliced √

½ cup chopped fresh parsley √

2 tablespoons sunflower seeds

1 teaspoon Dijon mustard

4 cups root vegetables, roasted √

1. Preheat the oven to 375°F. Line a sheet pan with parchment paper.

2. Roughly chop the cod and put the pieces in a large bowl. Add the egg, almond meal, red bell peppers, green onions, parsley, sunflower seeds, and mustard and stir to combine well.

3. Using your hands, shape the cod mixture into 4 patties, about 3 inches in diameter by 1 inch thick, and place on the prepared pan. Bake for 25 minutes, until golden brown on the surface and opaque and firm in the center.

4. Meanwhile, reheat the roasted root vegetables in the microwave or on the stovetop.

5. Divide the vegetables between two plates and top each plate with a cod cake. Store the remaining two cod cakes in the refrigerator for use in the Cod Cake Lettuce Wraps (page 71).

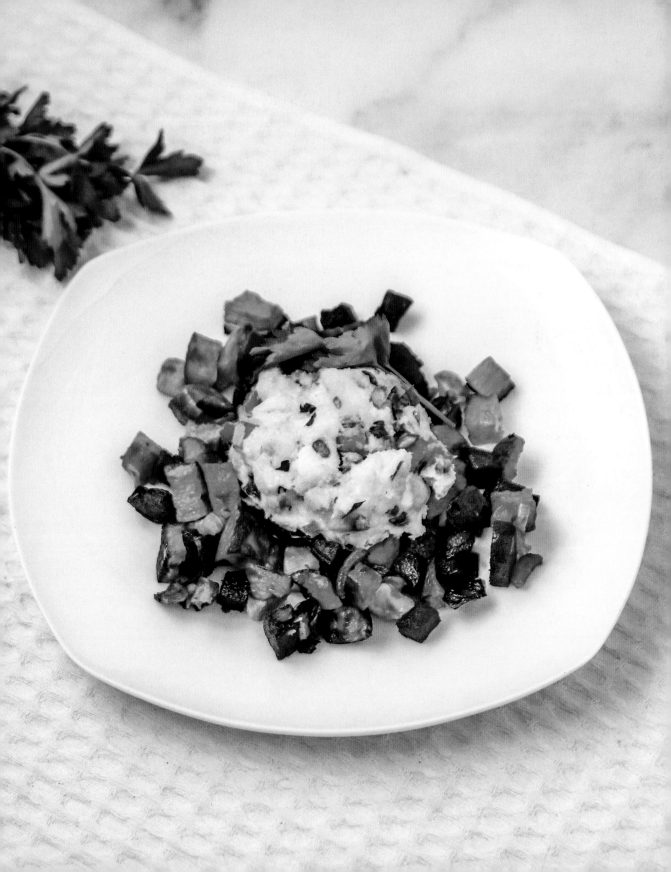

Week 4:

PORK, COCONUT OIL, APPLES, AND FLAXSEED

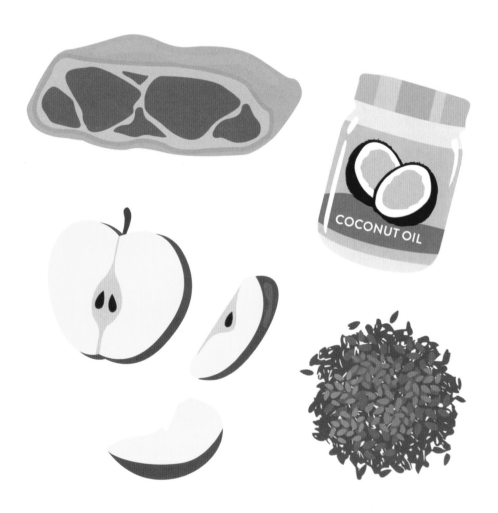

MENU

BREAKFAST	1	Apple-Flax Fiber Muffins
	2	Apple Pie Protein Oats
LUNCH	1	Pork Lettuce Cups
	2	Egg Roll Bowls
DINNER	1	One-Pan Flax-Crusted Pork Chops with Apple Slaw
	2	Pork Fried Rice

FEATURED INGREDIENTS

 ## PROTEIN

This week's featured protein is pork, which is a good source of nutrients important for PCOS, such as B vitamins and zinc. The recipes use both ground pork and pork chops. If you do not eat pork, feel free to substitute another protein, such as ground chicken, turkey, or beef.

 ## FIBER

Apples are this week's source of fiber. One medium apple contains approximately 5 grams of dietary fiber. Apples are also a good source of vitamin C and many antioxidants. You can use any type of apple you like in these recipes, such as McIntosh, Fuji, or Pink Lady.

 ## FAT

This week's fat is coconut oil. The fat in coconut oil is primarily saturated, but the type of saturated fat found in coconut oil is different from that found in animal products. Coconut oil is a good source of medium-chain triglycerides, which are processed differently in the body than other fats and may be beneficial for weight loss. Additionally, coconut oil adds a distinctive flavor to recipes. Depending on the temperature, coconut oil is solid at room temperature. It can also be purchased in liquid form.

 ## PCOS POWER FOOD

This week's PCOS Power Food is flaxseed. Flaxseed is high in anti-inflammatory omega-3 fatty acids and a type of fiber called lignans, which may help balance estrogen by binding to it in your intestines and helping your body eliminate it efficiently. One tablespoon of ground flaxseed contains 3 grams of healthy fats and 2 grams of fiber. Flaxseed can be used in recipes as a substitute for breadcrumbs or flour.

WEEKLY INGREDIENTS

FRESH PRODUCE

Apples (any type), 5

Bean sprouts, 2 cups

Carrot, 1

Cilantro, 1 bunch

Coleslaw mix, 4 cups

Garlic, 4 cloves

Ginger, 1 (3-inch) piece

Green beans, 12 ounces

Green leaf lettuce, 1 head

Green onions, 10

Red bell pepper, 1

Red cabbage, 1½ cups shredded

MEAT/SEAFOOD

Ground pork, 1½ pounds

Pork rib chops, bone-in, 2 (8 ounces each)

EGGS/DAIRY/MILK

Eggs, 4 large

Unsweetened nondairy milk of choice, 1 cup

SEASONINGS

Apple pie spice, 1 teaspoon

Chinese five-spice powder, 2 teaspoons (If you can't find Chinese five-spice, use 1 teaspoon ginger powder and 1 teaspoon garlic powder instead.)

Dried ground rosemary, 2 teaspoons

Ground cinnamon, 1 teaspoon

PANTRY

Apple cider vinegar, 2 tablespoons

Avocado oil, 1 tablespoon

Baking powder, 2 teaspoons

Brown rice, 1 cup

Chia seeds, 2 tablespoons

Chili paste, 2 teaspoons (optional, for Egg Roll Bowls)

Coconut oil, ½ cup

Collagen peptides or vanilla-flavored protein powder, 1 cup (8 scoops)

Cooking spray (avocado or olive oil)

Ground flaxseed, 1½ cups

Hemp seeds, hulled, 2 tablespoons

Honey, 1 teaspoon

Lemon juice, 1 tablespoon

Lime juice, 2 tablespoons

Old-fashioned oats, ½ cup

Peanuts, ¼ cup

Sesame oil, dark (toasted), 1 teaspoon

Tamari, ¼ cup plus 1 tablespoon

Vanilla extract, 2 teaspoons

Whole-grain mustard, 1 tablespoon

CUSTOMIZING THE PLAN

TO ADD MORE CARBS:

- Double the rice.
- Double the oats.
- Replace the riced cauliflower in the Pork Fried Rice with cooked brown rice.
- Use whole-grain wraps in place of the lettuce leaves in the Pork Lettuce Cups.

PREP DAY

Today you will be cooking the rice and ground pork and prepping some of the vegetables for the week. Prep the veggies while the rice and pork cook. Bake the Apple-Flax Fiber Muffins (page 81) and precook the Apple Pie Protein Oats (page 82) so you have them ready for the week.

Complete the following tasks and store each component in a separate container in the refrigerator for use later in the week.

COOK THE RICE

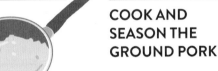

YIELD: 2 cups
PREP TIME: 2 minutes
COOK TIME: 25 minutes

Put 1 cup brown rice, 2 cups water, and ¼ teaspoon fine sea salt in a saucepan over medium-high heat. Bring to a boil, then lower the heat to medium, cover, and cook for 20 to 25 minutes, until all of the water is absorbed.

COOK AND SEASON THE GROUND PORK

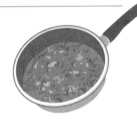

PREP TIME: 2 minutes
COOK TIME: 10 minutes

In a large skillet over medium-high heat, cook 1½ pounds ground pork until it is slightly browned and no longer pink, 10 to 15 minutes. Remove from the heat and stir in 2 teaspoons Chinese five-spice powder and 1 tablespoon tamari.

TRIM THE GREEN BEANS

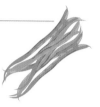

Trim the green beans and leave them whole.

SLICE THE GREEN ONIONS

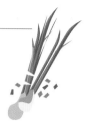

Thinly slice 10 green onions.

DICE THE RED BELL PEPPER

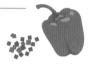

Dice enough red bell pepper to measure 1 cup.

CHOP THE CILANTRO

Finely chop enough cilantro to measure 1 cup.

SHRED THE RED CABBAGE

Shred enough red cabbage to measure 1½ cups. (If you bought preshredded cabbage, skip this step.)

MINCE THE GARLIC

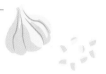

Mince 4 cloves of garlic.

MINCE THE GINGER

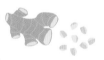

Peel and mince enough ginger to measure 3 tablespoons.

SHRED THE CARROT

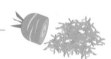

Shred enough carrot to measure ¼ cup.

Apple-Flax
FIBER MUFFINS

YIELD: 8 muffins (2 per serving)
PREP TIME: 5 minutes
COOK TIME: 20 minutes

1. Preheat the oven to 350°F and spray 8 wells of a standard-size muffin tin with cooking spray.

2. Grate the apples and squeeze out the excess water.

3. Put all of the ingredients in a large bowl and stir until well combined.

4. Divide the batter evenly among the greased wells of the muffin tin, filling them about two-thirds full.

5. Bake for 18 to 20 minutes, until a toothpick inserted in the middle of a muffin comes out clean. Remove from the oven, transfer the muffins to a cooling rack, and let cool.

6. Serve, or store in the refrigerator for later in the week.

2 apples (any type)

1¼ cups ground flaxseed

¾ cup collagen peptides or vanilla-flavored protein powder

2 teaspoons baking powder

1 teaspoon ground cinnamon

⅛ teaspoon fine sea salt

4 large eggs

¼ cup coconut oil, melted

1 teaspoon vanilla extract

NOTE:
These muffins freeze well, so you can freeze any leftovers that you do not plan on eating within the week.

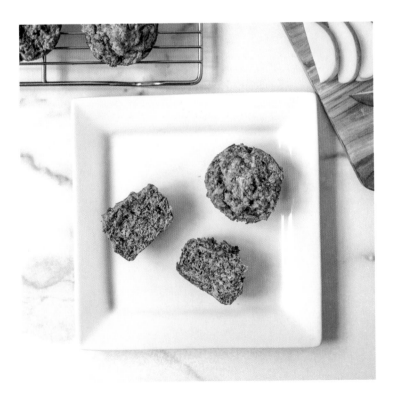

Apple Pie
PROTEIN OATS

YIELD: 2 servings
PREP TIME: 3 minutes
COOK TIME: 8 minutes

½ cup old-fashioned oats

1 cup unsweetened nondairy milk of choice

2 tablespoons chia seeds

2 tablespoons hulled hemp seeds

1 apple (any type)

¼ cup (2 scoops) vanilla-flavored protein powder or collagen peptides

2 tablespoons ground flaxseed

1 teaspoon apple pie spice (or a mixture of allspice, cinnamon, and nutmeg)

1 teaspoon vanilla extract

1. Put the oats, milk, chia seeds, and hemp seeds in a small saucepan over medium heat and cook, stirring frequently, until the milk is absorbed, about 5 minutes.

2. Finely dice the apple and add it to the pot with the oats. Stir to combine, then cook until the apple is warmed through, about 3 minutes.

3. Remove from the heat and stir in the protein powder, flaxseed, apple pie spice, and vanilla.

4. Serve, or store in the refrigerator for later in the week.

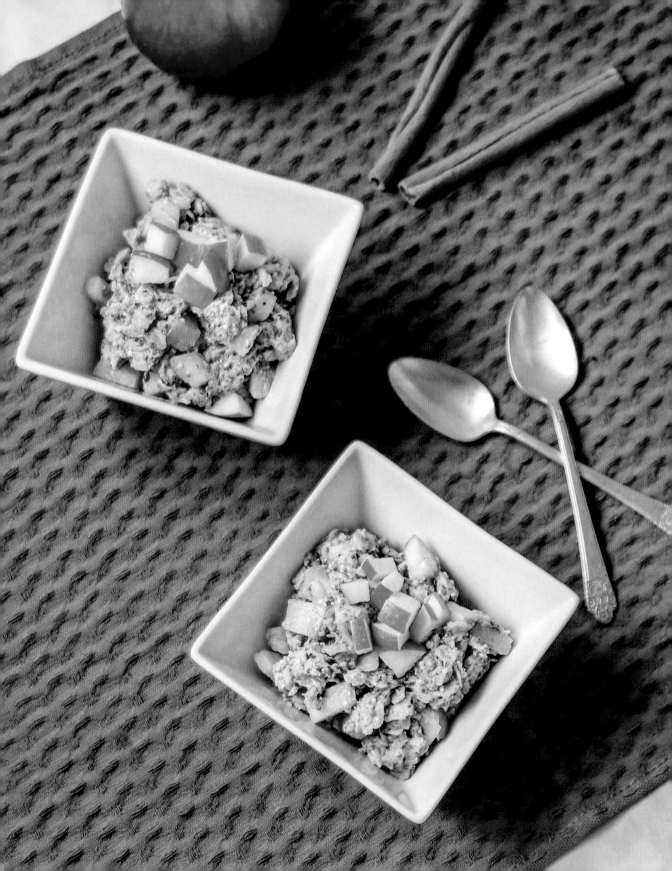

YIELD: 2 servings
PREP TIME: 5 minutes
COOK TIME: —

Pork
LETTUCE CUPS

4 leaves green lettuce

2 tablespoons tamari

1 tablespoon lime juice

2 teaspoons coconut oil, melted

1 clove garlic, minced √

1 teaspoon minced ginger √

One-third of the cooked and seasoned ground pork √

½ cup shredded red cabbage √

¼ cup shredded carrots √

2 green onions, thinly sliced √

½ cup chopped fresh cilantro √

¼ cup peanuts

1. Place two lettuce leaves on each of two plates.

2. Make the dressing: In a small bowl, whisk together the tamari, lime juice, coconut oil, garlic, and ginger.

3. Top the lettuce leaves with the cooked pork, cabbage, carrots, green onions, cilantro, and peanuts. Drizzle with the dressing.

4. Serve, or store in the refrigerator for later in the week.

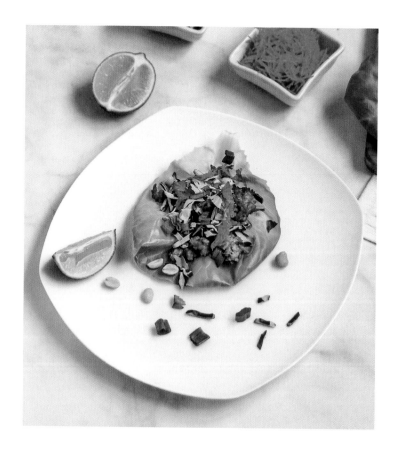

Egg Roll
BOWLS

YIELD: 2 servings
PREP TIME: 5 minutes
COOK TIME: 5 minutes

1. Heat the oil in a large skillet. Add the coleslaw mix, bean sprouts, green onions, garlic, ginger, and tamari. Cook, stirring, until the cabbage is softened, about 2 minutes.

2. Add the pork and cook until heated through, about 3 minutes.

3. Serve with the rice and top with the chili paste, if desired.

4. Serve, or store in the refrigerator for later in the week.

1 tablespoon coconut oil

4 cups coleslaw mix

2 cups bean sprouts

4 green onions, thinly sliced √

2 cloves garlic, minced √

1 tablespoon minced ginger √

1 tablespoon tamari

One-third of the cooked and seasoned ground pork √

1 cup cooked brown rice √

2 teaspoons chili paste (optional)

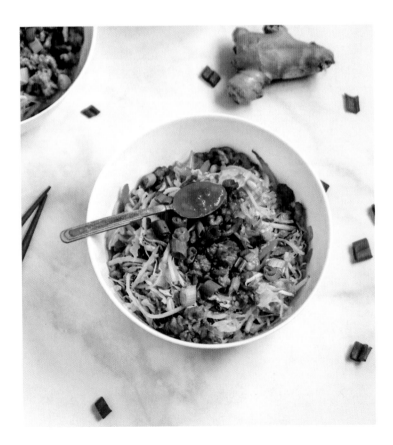

One-Pan Flax-Crusted Pork Chops with APPLE SLAW

YIELD: 2 servings
PREP TIME: 10 minutes
COOK TIME: 25 minutes

2 (8-ounce) bone-in pork rib chops

1 tablespoon coconut oil

2 tablespoons apple cider vinegar, divided

1 tablespoon ground flaxseed

1 tablespoon whole-grain mustard

2 teaspoons ground dried rosemary

Salt and pepper

2 cups green beans, trimmed √

2 apples (any type)

1 cup shredded red cabbage √

2 green onions, thinly sliced √

1 tablespoon avocado oil

1 tablespoon lemon juice

1 teaspoon honey

1. Preheat the oven to 400°F and line a sheet pan with parchment paper.

2. Place the pork chops in the center of the prepared pan.

3. Put the coconut oil, 1 tablespoon of the vinegar, the flaxseed, mustard, and rosemary in a small bowl and whisk to combine. Season with salt and pepper. Spread the mixture over the pork chops.

4. Arrange the green beans on the sheet pan surrounding the pork chops and bake for 25 minutes, or until the chops are cooked through.

5. Meanwhile, make the slaw: Grate the apples and squeeze out the excess liquid. Put the apples in a large bowl. Add the cabbage, green onions, avocado oil, lemon juice, honey, and remaining tablespoon of vinegar and toss to combine. Season with salt and pepper to taste.

6. Divide the pork chops and green beans between two plates and serve the apple slaw on the side, or store the components separately for later in the week.

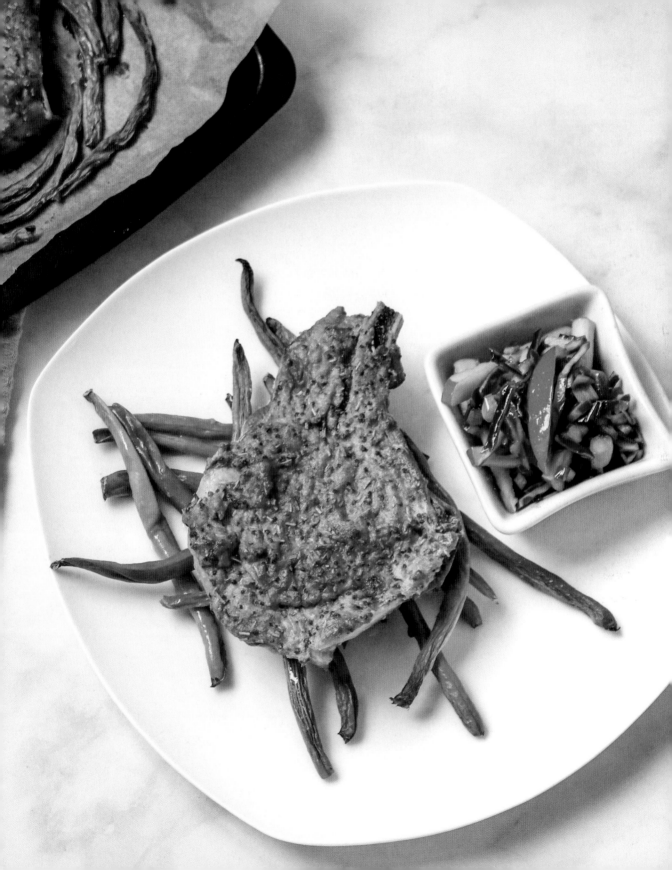

YIELD: 2 servings
PREP TIME: 5 minutes
COOK TIME: 10 minutes

Pork
FRIED RICE

1 cup frozen peas

½ cup frozen riced cauliflower

1 tablespoon coconut oil

2 green onions, thinly sliced √

1 cup diced red bell peppers √

1 clove garlic, minced √

1 tablespoon minced ginger √

One-third of the cooked and
seasoned ground pork √

1 cup cooked brown rice √

1 tablespoon tamari

1 teaspoon dark (toasted)
sesame oil

½ cup chopped fresh cilantro

1 tablespoon lime juice

1. In a large skillet, sauté the frozen peas and riced cauliflower in the coconut oil over medium-high heat until fully thawed, about 5 minutes.

2. Add the green onions, red bell peppers, garlic, and ginger and cook for 2 minutes, until the onions and peppers are slightly softened.

3. Add the pork, brown rice, tamari, and sesame oil to the pan and cook until warmed through, about 3 minutes.

4. Stir in the cilantro and lime juice and serve, or store in the refrigerator for later in the week.

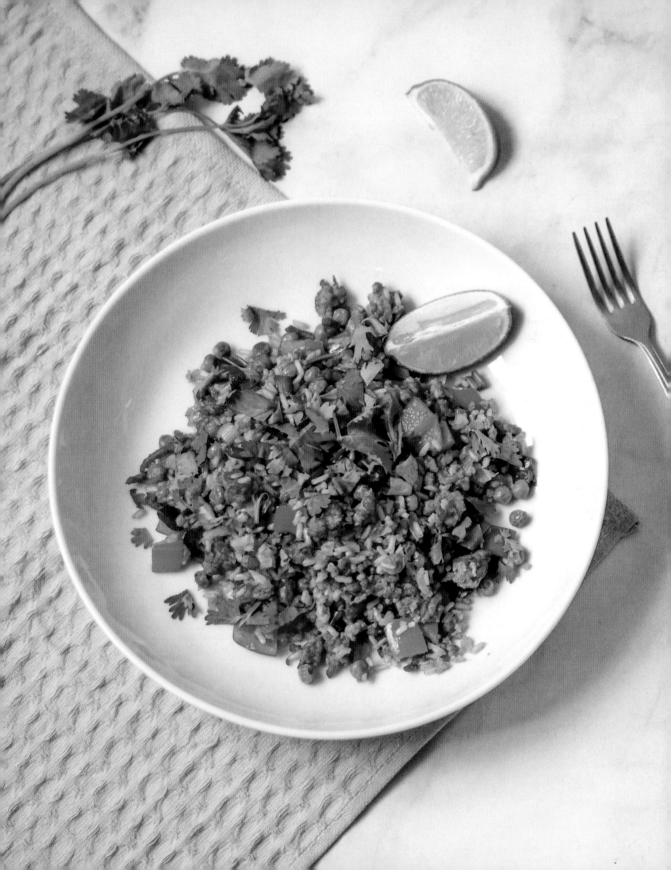

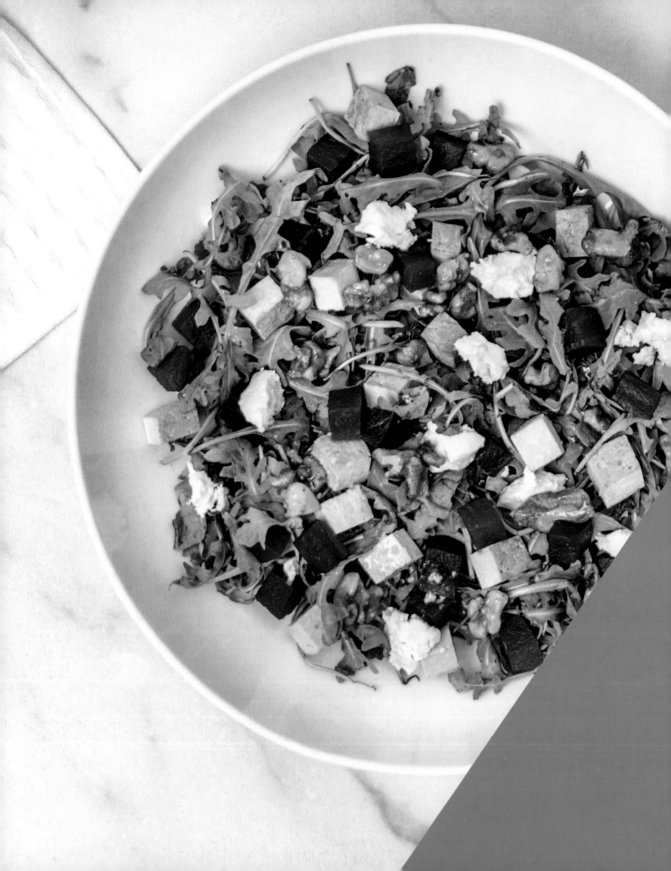

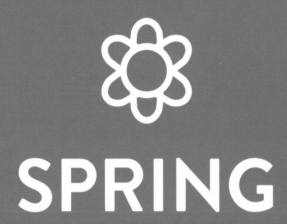

SPRING

Week 5:

SALMON, AVOCADO, WHITE BEANS, AND ARTICHOKE HEARTS

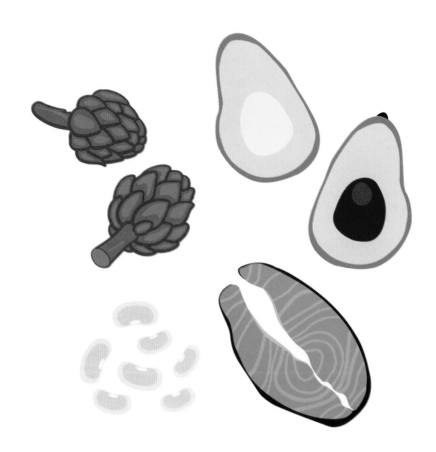

MENU

BREAKFAST	1	High-Protein Grain Bowls
	2	Mediterranean Omelette
LUNCH	1	Salmon-Stuffed Avocado Cups
	2	Salmon Poke Bowl
DINNER	1	White Bean Cakes with Artichoke Quinoa Pilaf
	2	Paprika Salmon with Garlic Quinoa

FEATURED INGREDIENTS

 ### PROTEIN

This week's featured protein is salmon, which is high in protein and healthy anti-inflammatory omega-3 fats. The recipes for this week use both fresh and smoked salmon. If you are watching your sodium levels or do not wish to consume smoked salmon, you may substitute cooked fresh salmon for the smoked salmon in these recipes.

 ### FIBER

White beans are this week's main source of fiber. One cup of cooked white beans contains 47 grams of carbohydrates, 19 grams of which are fiber, making them a smart carb choice for PCOS. They also add plant-based protein, with 15 grams per cup. Additionally, they are high in magnesium, which is a common nutrient deficiency in women with PCOS.

 ### FAT

This week's fat is avocado, which is not only a good source of monounsaturated fats but also high in fiber. Avocados brown quickly after cutting, so they should not be prepped in advance.

 ### PCOS POWER FOOD

This week's PCOS Power Food is artichoke hearts. Artichokes are one of the highest-fiber foods available, with 6 grams of fiber per 1 cup of hearts. The recipes call for quartered artichoke hearts in water, which you can find in the canned vegetable aisle. Some stores sell frozen artichoke hearts as well. Do not use marinated artichoke hearts in these recipes, as many are made with inflammatory vegetable oils, and their flavor may not blend well in the recipes.

WEEKLY INGREDIENTS

FRESH PRODUCE

Arugula, 3 cups

Avocados, Hass, 3

Cherry tomatoes, 1 pint

Cucumbers, 3

Garlic, 8 cloves

Green onions, 1 bunch

Parsley, curly or Italian, 1 bunch

Red bell pepper, 1

Shallots, 2 medium

Spinach, 2 cups

Yellow onion, 1

MEAT/SEAFOOD

Salmon fillets, 4 (4 ounces each)

Smoked salmon, 8 ounces

EGGS/DAIRY/MILK

Eggs, 13 large

Feta cheese, ¼ cup crumbled (optional, for egg scramble)

Unsweetened nondairy milk of choice, 2 tablespoons

PANTRY

Almond flour, blanched, ½ cup

Artichoke hearts, quartered, 3 (14-ounce) cans

Cooking spray (avocado or olive oil)

Dijon mustard, 1 tablespoon

Kalamata olives, pitted, ½ cup

Lemon juice, ½ cup

Olive oil, extra-virgin, ¼ cup plus 2 tablespoons

Quinoa, 2 cups

Rice vinegar, 1 tablespoon

Sesame seeds, 1 tablespoon

Sushi nori, 1 sheet

Tamari, 1 tablespoon

White beans, 1½ cups dried or 2 (15-ounce) cans

SEASONINGS

Dried oregano, 1 teaspoon

Smoked paprika, 1 teaspoon

CUSTOMIZING THE PLAN

TO ADD MORE CARBS:

- Double the quinoa.
- Double the beans.
- Have a piece of whole-grain toast with the Mediterranean Omelette.

PREP DAY

Today you will be cooking the quinoa, beans, and some of the salmon and eggs and prepping some of the vegetables for the week. Start with the quinoa, beans, and salmon and prep the eggs and veggies while they cook.

Complete the following tasks and store each component in a separate container in the refrigerator for use later in the week.

COOK THE QUINOA

YIELD: about 2 cups
PREP TIME: 2 minutes
COOK TIME: 20 minutes

Put 2 cups quinoa, 4 cups water, and ½ teaspoon fine sea salt in a stockpot over medium-high heat. Bring to a boil, then lower the heat to medium and cover. Cook until all of the water is absorbed, about 20 minutes.

COOK THE BEANS

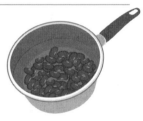

YIELD: 3 cups
PREP TIME: 2 minutes
COOK TIME: 1 hour

If using dried beans, place 1½ cups beans and 4½ cups water in a large saucepan. Bring to a boil, then lower the heat to a simmer and cover. Cook until the beans are soft, about 1 hour, then stir in ½ teaspoon fine sea salt. If you purchased canned beans, you can rinse them and place them in a storage container.

BAKE SOME OF THE SALMON

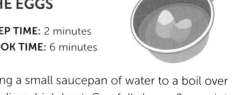

PREP TIME: 1 minute
COOK TIME: 20 minutes

Preheat the oven to 375°F. Line a sheet pan with parchment paper or spray it with cooking spray. Place two 4-ounce salmon fillets on the prepared pan and season with salt and pepper. Bake for 20 minutes, or until the salmon is opaque in the center.

SOFT-BOIL SOME OF THE EGGS

PREP TIME: 2 minutes
COOK TIME: 6 minutes

Bring a small saucepan of water to a boil over medium-high heat. Carefully lower 2 eggs into the water and reduce the heat to a simmer. After 6 minutes, remove the eggs from the pan and place in a bowl of cold water for 10 minutes. When the eggs are cool, peel them.

SLICE THE GREEN ONIONS

Thinly slice 6 green onions.

SLICE THE YELLOW ONION

Thinly slice enough yellow onion to measure ½ cup.

SLICE THE SHALLOTS

Thinly slice enough shallots to measure ½ cup.

SLICE THE RED BELL PEPPER

Thinly slice enough red bell pepper to measure ½ cup.

SLICE AND DICE THE CUCUMBER

Slice enough cucumber to measure 3 cups and dice enough cucumber to measure 1 cup. Store the sliced and diced cucumbers separately.

CHOP THE PARSLEY

Finely chop enough fresh parsley to measure 1 cup.

MINCE THE GARLIC

Mince 8 cloves of garlic.

HALVE THE TOMATOES

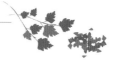

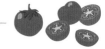

Halve 1 pint of cherry tomatoes.

High-Protein
GRAIN BOWLS

YIELD: 2 servings
PREP TIME: 5 minutes
COOK TIME: —

1. Peel the eggs and cut them in half.

2. In two bowls, arrange the quinoa, beans, cucumbers, artichoke hearts, smoked salmon, and eggs.

3. Drizzle with the oil and season with salt and pepper to taste.

4. Serve, or store in the refrigerator for later in the week.

1 cup cooked quinoa √

1 cup cooked white beans √

1 cup diced cucumbers √

1 cup quartered artichoke hearts, drained

4 ounces smoked salmon

2 soft-boiled eggs √

1 tablespoon extra-virgin olive oil

Salt and pepper

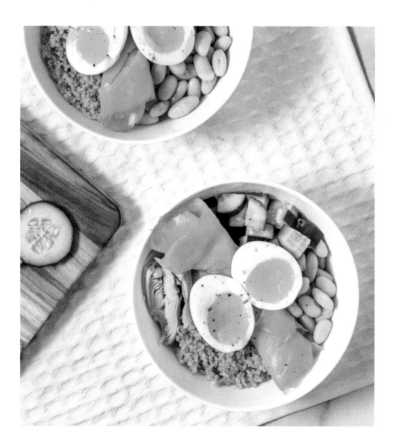

Mediterranean
OMELETTE

YIELD: 2 servings
PREP TIME: 5 minutes
COOK TIME: 15 minutes

½ cup sliced yellow onions √

½ cup sliced red bell peppers √

1 tablespoon extra-virgin olive oil

4 large eggs

6 large egg whites

2 tablespoons unsweetened nondairy milk of choice

Salt and pepper

1 cup quartered artichoke hearts, drained

1 cup cherry tomatoes, halved √

¼ cup pitted Kalamata olives

2 cloves garlic, minced √

1 teaspoon dried oregano leaves

¼ cup crumbled feta cheese (optional)

1. In a large skillet, sauté the onions and bell peppers in the oil over medium-high heat until soft, about 5 minutes.

2. Meanwhile, in a medium bowl, whisk the whole eggs and egg whites with the milk and season with salt and pepper.

3. Spray a small skillet with cooking spray. Pour in half of the egg mixture and cook over medium heat until the top is set. Remove from the pan and place on a plate.

4. Cook the remaining egg mixture in the same skillet and place on a second plate.

5. Add the artichoke hearts, tomatoes, olives, garlic, and oregano to the skillet with the onions and peppers and cook until heated through, about 3 minutes.

6. Scoop half of the vegetable mixture onto one half of each omelette. Fold the other half of the eggs over the vegetables. Sprinkle with the feta cheese, if using.

7. Serve, or store in the refrigerator for later in the week.

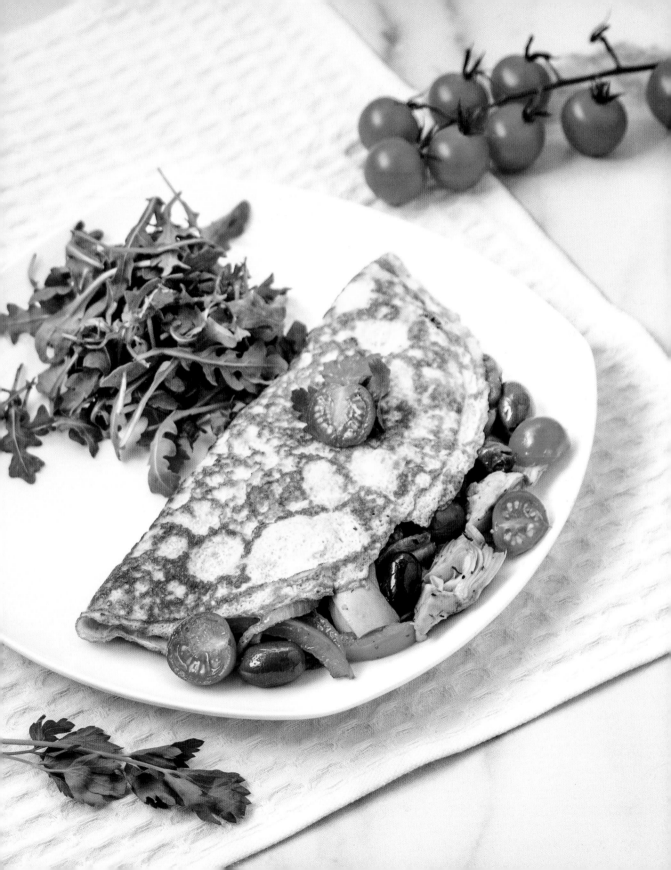

Salmon-Stuffed
AVOCADO CUPS

YIELD: 2 servings
PREP TIME: 5 minutes
COOK TIME: —

2 (4-ounce) salmon fillets, baked √

2 tablespoons lemon juice

1 tablespoon Dijon mustard

2 green onions, thinly sliced √

Salt and pepper

2 Hass avocados

2 cups sliced cucumbers √

1. In a medium bowl, mash the salmon with the lemon juice and mustard using a fork, then stir in the green onions. Season with salt and pepper to taste.

2. Slice the avocados in half and remove the pits.

3. Stuff the salmon mixture into the avocado halves and serve with the cucumber slices on the side.

4. Eat immediately, or store in the refrigerator for later in the week.

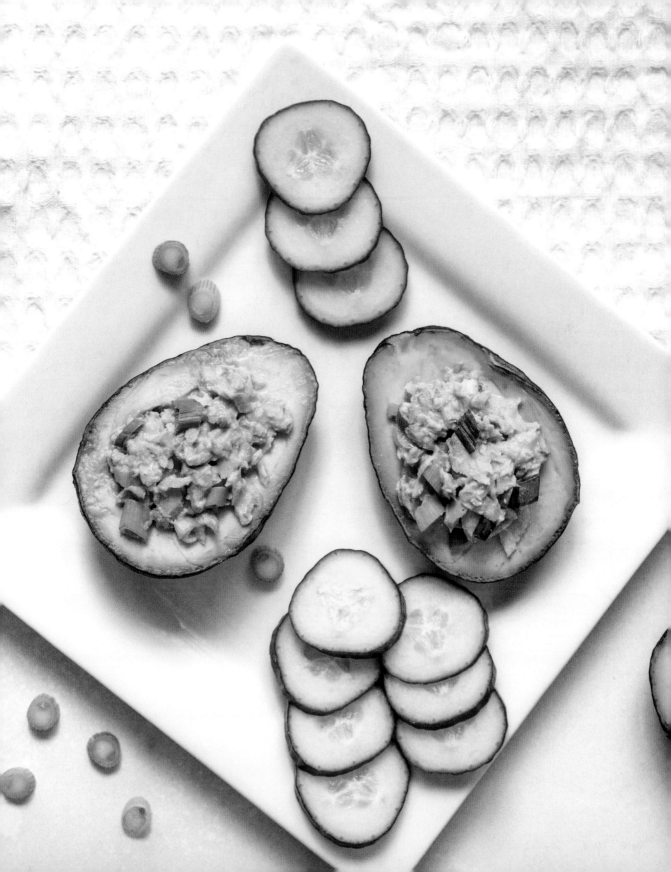

YIELD: 2 servings
PREP TIME: 5 minutes
COOK TIME: —

Salmon
POKE BOWL

1 cup cooked quinoa √

1 tablespoon rice vinegar

1 tablespoon tamari

3 cups arugula

1 cup sliced cucumbers √

4 ounces smoked salmon

½ Hass avocado

1 sheet sushi nori

2 green onions, thinly sliced √

1 tablespoon black or white sesame seeds

1. Put the quinoa, vinegar, and tamari in a medium bowl and mix well.

2. Divide the arugula evenly between two serving bowls. Top with the quinoa mixture, cucumbers, and smoked salmon.

3. Slice the avocado and divide it between the bowls.

4. Using kitchen scissors, cut the nori into thin strips and divide it between the bowls.

5. Sprinkle the green onions and sesame seeds over the bowls.

6. Serve, or store in the refrigerator for later in the week.

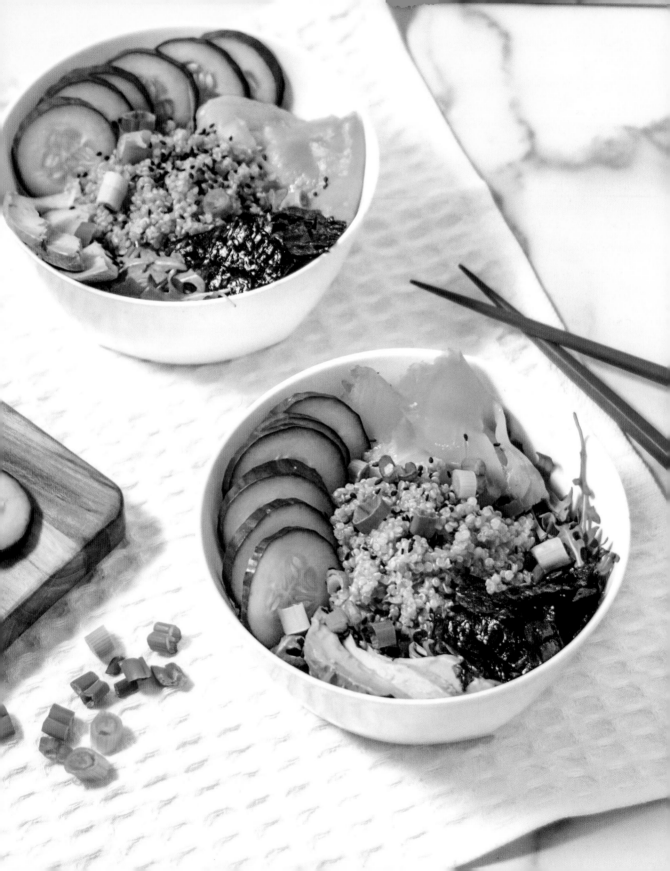

White Bean Cakes with
ARTICHOKE QUINOA PILAF

YIELD: 2 servings
PREP TIME: 10 minutes
COOK TIME: 25 minutes

1 cup cooked white beans √

2 green onions, thinly sliced √

1 large egg

½ cup blanched almond flour

Salt and pepper

2 tablespoons extra-virgin olive oil

1 cup cooked quinoa √

2 cloves garlic, minced √

1 cup quartered artichoke hearts, drained

½ cup chopped fresh parsley

¼ cup pitted Kalamata olives

2 tablespoons lemon juice

NOTE:
The white bean cakes freeze well, so you can freeze any that you don't plan on eating within the week.

1. Preheat the oven to 375°F and line a sheet pan with parchment paper.

2. Make the bean cakes: In a medium bowl, combine the beans, green onions, egg, and almond flour, mashing the beans lightly with a fork. Season with salt and pepper. Shape into two cakes and place on the prepared pan. Bake for 20 minutes, flipping the cakes over carefully halfway through cooking, until golden brown on both sides.

3. Meanwhile, make the pilaf: Heat the oil in a large skillet over medium-high heat. Add the quinoa and garlic and cook, stirring, for about 3 minutes, until warmed through. Add the artichoke hearts, parsley, olives, and lemon juice and cook until heated through, about 3 minutes. Season with salt and pepper to taste.

4. Divide the quinoa mixture between two plates and top with the bean cakes, or store the components separately for later in the week.

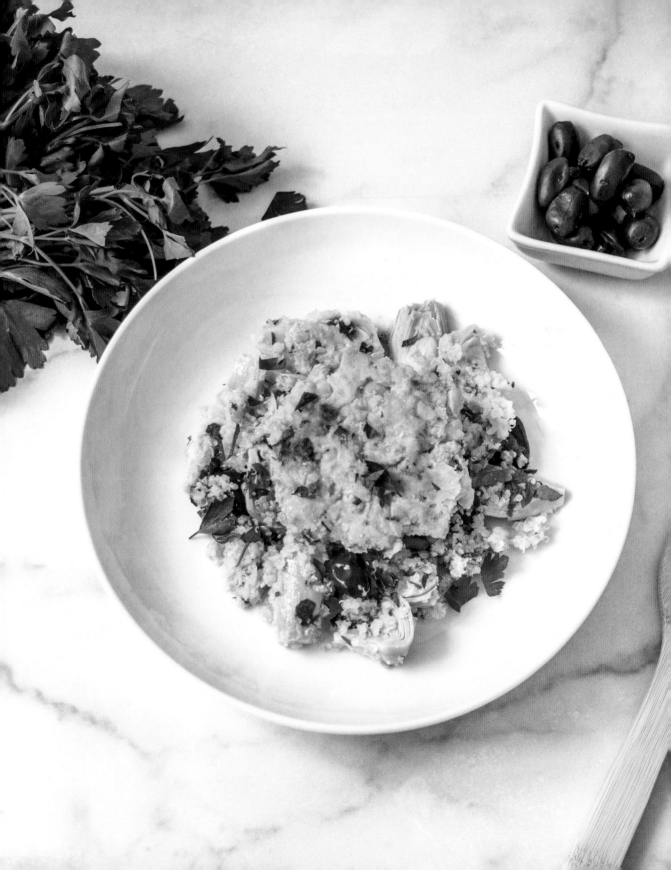

YIELD: 2 servings
PREP TIME: 5 minutes
COOK TIME: 10 minutes

Paprika Salmon with
GARLIC QUINOA

½ cup thinly sliced shallots √

4 cloves garlic, minced, divided √

2 tablespoons extra-virgin olive oil, divided

2 (4-ounce) salmon fillets

1 cup quartered artichoke hearts, drained

1 cup cherry tomatoes, halved √

¼ cup lemon juice

1 teaspoon smoked paprika

1 cup cooked quinoa √

2 cups fresh spinach

1 cup cooked white beans √

½ cup chopped fresh parsley √

1. In a medium skillet, sauté the shallots and 2 cloves of the garlic in 1 tablespoon of the oil over medium-high heat until the shallots are softened.

2. Add the salmon, artichoke hearts, tomatoes, lemon juice, and smoked paprika, reduce the heat to low, and cover. Cook until the fish is opaque in the center, about 10 minutes.

3. Meanwhile, in a large skillet, heat the remaining tablespoon of oil over medium-high heat. Add the quinoa and the remaining 2 cloves of garlic and cook, stirring, for about 3 minutes, until warmed through.

4. Roughly chop the spinach, then add it to the pan with the quinoa, along with the beans and parsley. Cook until the spinach is wilted, about 3 minutes.

5. Divide the quinoa mixture between two plates and top with the salmon and vegetables, or store the components separately for later in the week.

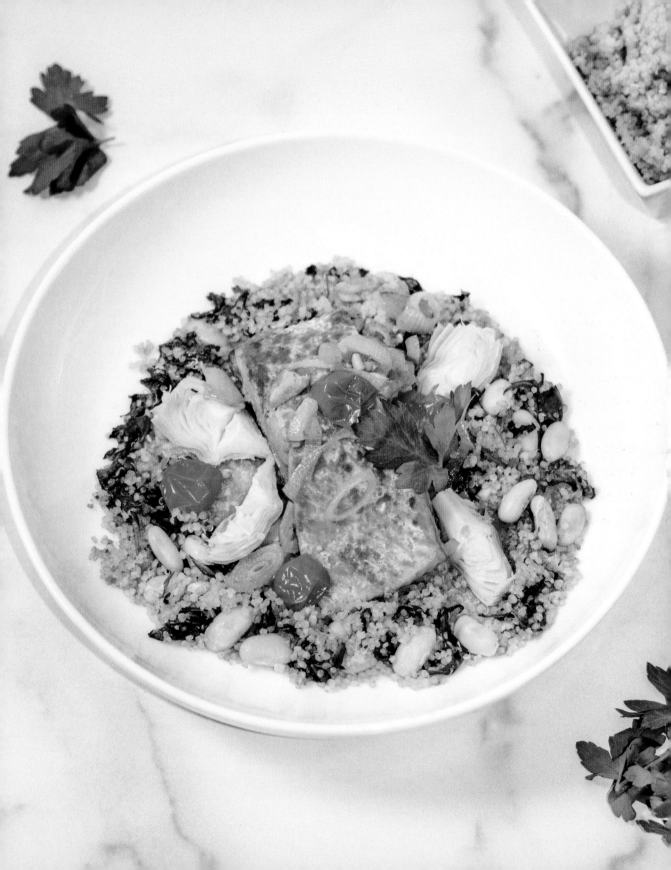

Week 6:

TOFU, WALNUTS, BLACK BEANS, AND BEETS

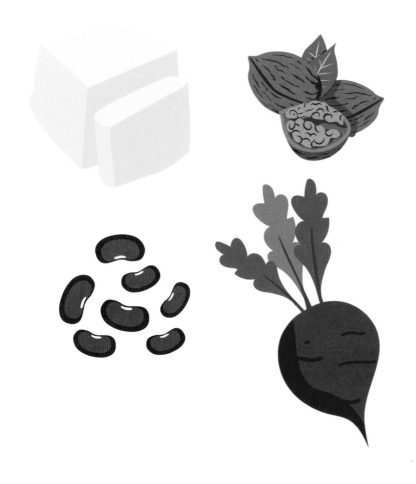

MENU

BREAKFAST	1	Tofu Scramble
	2	Black Bean Chocolate Walnut Muffins
LUNCH	1	Beet Salad with Goat Cheese and Spiced Walnuts
	2	High-Protein Black Bean Soup
DINNER	1	Black Bean Enchiladas
	2	Black Bean Beet Burgers with Roasted Spring Veggies

FEATURED INGREDIENTS

PROTEIN

This week's featured protein is tofu. There's a lot of misinformation out there about soy because it contains phytoestrogens (plant-based estrogenlike compounds), but phytoestrogens have a much weaker action compared to our bodies' own estrogens, and evidence shows that consuming soy actually protects against breast cancer. Soy is one of the highest-protein plant foods available. I recommend purchasing organic tofu if you are concerned about avoiding GMOs and pesticides.

FAT

This week's fat is walnuts, which are high in anti-inflammatory omega-3 fatty acids. They are also a good source of magnesium and B vitamins, both of which are beneficial for PCOS.

FIBER

Black beans are this week's main source of fiber. One cup of cooked black beans contains 15 grams of fiber, along with 15 grams of protein. Although they are high in carbohydrates, beans are a smart carb choice for PCOS. Additionally, they are high in magnesium, which is a common nutrient deficiency in PCOS, as well as a good source of iron and B vitamins.

PCOS POWER FOOD

This week's PCOS Power Food is beets. Beets are low in calories and are a good source of many beneficial compounds for PCOS. For example, betalains may help reduce inflammation, and dietary nitrates may help lower blood pressure. Additionally, beets contain fibers that are beneficial to gut health. Cooking beets from scratch is the most affordable method, but if you're short on time, you can purchase them already cooked in the produce section of most grocery stores.

WEEKLY INGREDIENTS

FRESH PRODUCE

Arugula, 4 cups

Asparagus, 1 bundle

Beets, 3 medium

Cilantro, 1 bunch

Garlic, 7 cloves

Green bell peppers, 2

Jalapeño pepper, 1

Parsley, curly or Italian, 1 bunch

Red bell peppers, 2

Shiitake mushrooms, 4 ounces

Spinach, 4 cups

Yellow onions, 3

MEAT/SEAFOOD

Extra-firm tofu, 1½ pounds

Firm tofu, 1 pound

EGGS/DAIRY/MILK

Eggs, 5 large

Goat cheese, 2 ounces (optional, for beet salad)

Shredded Mexican cheese blend, ¼ cup (optional, for enchiladas)

PANTRY

Apple cider vinegar, 1 tablespoon

Avocado oil, 2 tablespoons

Baking powder, 1 teaspoon

Black beans, 2½ cups dried or 4 (15-ounce) cans

Bone broth, chicken or beef, 2 cups

Cacao powder or cocoa powder, ⅓ cup

Chickpea flour, ½ cup

Coconut sugar, ¼ cup

Cooking spray (avocado or olive oil)

Dijon mustard, 2 teaspoons

Ground flaxseed, 2 tablespoons

Lemon juice, 1 tablespoon

Lime juice, 2 tablespoons

Low-carb whole-wheat wraps, 4

Maple syrup, 1 tablespoon

Olive oil, extra-virgin, ½ cup

Protein powder, unflavored or vanilla-flavored, ¼ cup

Tamari, 1 tablespoon

Tomato paste, 1 tablespoon

Tomatoes, whole peeled, 1 (15-ounce) can

Walnuts, raw, 1¼ cups

SEASONINGS

Chili powder, 1 tablespoon

Ground cinnamon, ½ teaspoon

Turmeric powder, ½ teaspoon

Vanilla extract, 1 teaspoon

CUSTOMIZING THE PLAN

TO ADD MORE CARBS:

Because this week is plant-based, it's already a little higher in carbs than the other weeks. But if you need even more carbs:

- Double the beets.
- Double the beans.
- Have a piece of whole-grain toast with the Tofu Scramble.

TO MAKE THIS WEEK DAIRY-FREE:

- Omit the cheeses.

PREP DAY

Today you will be cooking the beets, beans, and tofu, toasting the walnuts, making the salsa, and prepping some of the vegetables. Start with the beets and beans and prep the walnuts, tofu, salsa, and veggies while they cook. Also bake the Black Bean Chocolate Walnut Muffins (page 116).

Complete the following tasks and store each component in a separate container in the refrigerator for use later in the week.

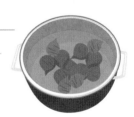

COOK AND PREP THE BEETS

YIELD: 2 cups
PREP TIME: 5 minutes
COOK TIME: 45 to 60 minutes

If using fresh beets, place 3 whole beets in a stockpot. Cover with water and add 1 tablespoon apple cider vinegar and ½ teaspoon fine sea salt. Cover and bring to a boil. Reduce the heat to a simmer and cook until the beets are tender (use a fork to check), 45 to 60 minutes. Watch the water carefully so that it doesn't boil off. Once the beets are cooked, immediately transfer to a bowl of cold water. When they are cool enough to handle, rub off the skins with your hands and dice enough beets to measure 1½ cups.

COOK THE BEANS

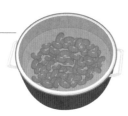

YIELD: 5 cups
PREP TIME: 2 minutes
COOK TIME: 1 hour

Put 2½ cups dried black beans and 7½ cups water in a stockpot. Bring to a boil, then reduce the heat to a simmer and cover. Cook until the beans are soft, about 1 hour, then stir in ½ teaspoon fine sea salt. If you purchased canned beans, you can rinse them and place them in a storage container.

BAKE SOME OF THE TOFU

PREP TIME: 1 minute
COOK TIME: 20 minutes

Preheat the oven to 375°F and line a sheet pan with parchment paper. Drain and cube 8 ounces extra-firm tofu and place it on the prepared pan. Sprinkle with 1 tablespoon tamari and bake for 20 minutes, turning the cubes over halfway through baking, until golden brown.

TOAST AND SPICE SOME OF THE WALNUTS

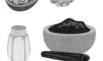

PREP TIME: 2 minutes
COOK TIME: 5 minutes

Preheat the oven to 200°F and line a sheet pan with parchment paper. Toss ½ cup raw walnuts with 2 teaspoons maple syrup, ½ teaspoon ground cinnamon, and ⅛ teaspoon fine sea salt and spread in an even layer on the prepared pan. Bake for 8 to 10 minutes, until lightly toasted, watching carefully so the nuts don't burn. Store in an airtight jar.

DICE THE ONION

Dice enough yellow onion to measure 2 cups. Set aside ¼ cup for the salsa and store the rest for use later in the week.

CHOP THE CILANTRO

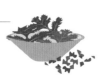

Finely chop enough fresh cilantro to measure ¼ cup and set aside for the salsa.

DICE THE JALAPEÑO

Dice 1 jalapeño pepper and remove the seeds, if desired. Set aside for the salsa.

MAKE THE SALSA

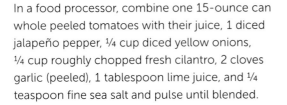

YIELD: about 2 cups
PREP TIME: 2 minutes
COOK TIME: —

In a food processor, combine one 15-ounce can whole peeled tomatoes with their juice, 1 diced jalapeño pepper, ¼ cup diced yellow onions, ¼ cup roughly chopped fresh cilantro, 2 cloves garlic (peeled), 1 tablespoon lime juice, and ¼ teaspoon fine sea salt and pulse until blended.

DICE THE BELL PEPPERS

Dice enough red and green bell peppers to measure 1 cup each.

MINCE THE REMAINING GARLIC

Mince 5 cloves of garlic.

TRIM AND CHOP THE ASPARAGUS

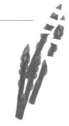

Trim and discard the tough ends off the asparagus and chop it into 1-inch pieces.

CHOP THE SPINACH

Chop enough fresh spinach to measure 4 cups.

SLICE THE MUSHROOMS

Slice enough shiitake mushrooms to measure 1 cup.

CHOP THE PARSLEY

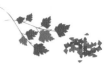

Finely chop enough fresh parsley to measure ½ cup.

YIELD: 2 servings
PREP TIME: 5 minutes
COOK TIME: 5 minutes

Tofu
SCRAMBLE

½ cup diced yellow onions √

½ cup diced green bell peppers √

1 tablespoon extra-virgin olive oil

1 pound firm tofu

½ cup cooked black beans √

1 tablespoon tomato paste

1 clove garlic, minced √

1 teaspoon chili powder

½ teaspoon turmeric powder

Salt and pepper

1. In a large skillet, sauté the onions and bell peppers in the oil over medium-high heat until soft, about 3 minutes.

2. Drain and crumble the tofu and add it to the pan. Add the beans, tomato paste, garlic, chili powder, turmeric, and salt and pepper to taste and cook until heated through, about 2 minutes.

3. Serve, or store in the refrigerator for later in the week.

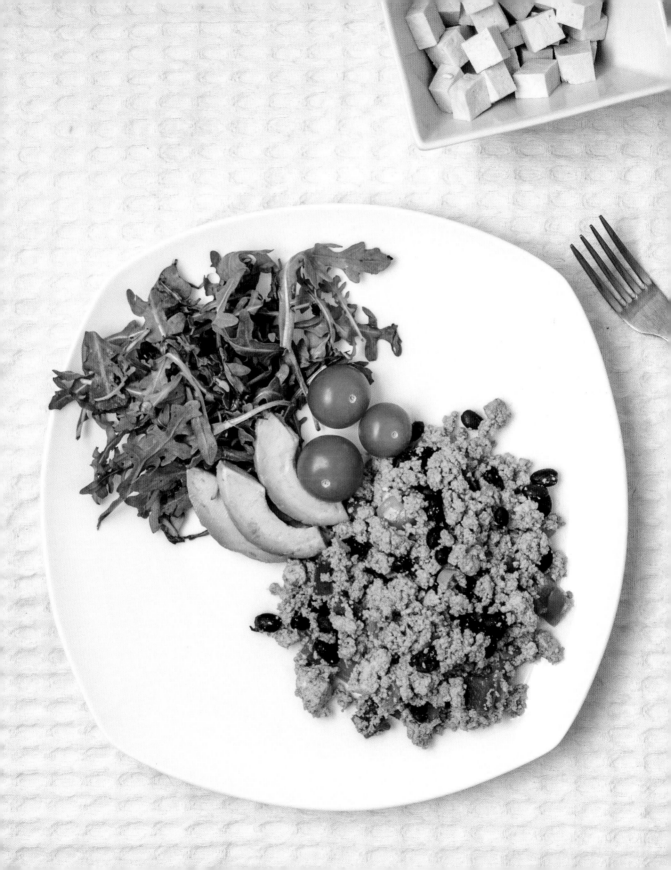

YIELD: 8 muffins (2 per serving)
PREP TIME: 10 minutes
COOK TIME: 25 minutes

Black Bean Chocolate
WALNUT MUFFINS

1½ cups cooked black beans √

4 large eggs

2 tablespoons avocado oil

1 teaspoon vanilla extract

⅓ cup cacao powder or cocoa powder

¼ cup coconut sugar

¼ cup unflavored or vanilla-flavored protein powder

2 tablespoons ground flaxseed

1 teaspoon baking powder

⅛ teaspoon fine sea salt

½ cup raw walnuts

1. Preheat the oven to 350°F and spray 8 wells of a standard-size muffin tin with cooking spray.

2. Put all of the ingredients except the walnuts in a food processor and process until smooth. Stir in the walnuts by hand.

3. Pour the batter evenly into the greased wells of the muffin tin, filling them about two-thirds full. Bake for 22 to 25 minutes, until a toothpick inserted in the center of a muffin comes out clean.

4. Remove from the oven, transfer the muffins to a cooling rack, and let cool. Serve, or store for later in the week.

NOTE:
These muffins freeze well, so you can freeze any that you don't plan on eating within the week.

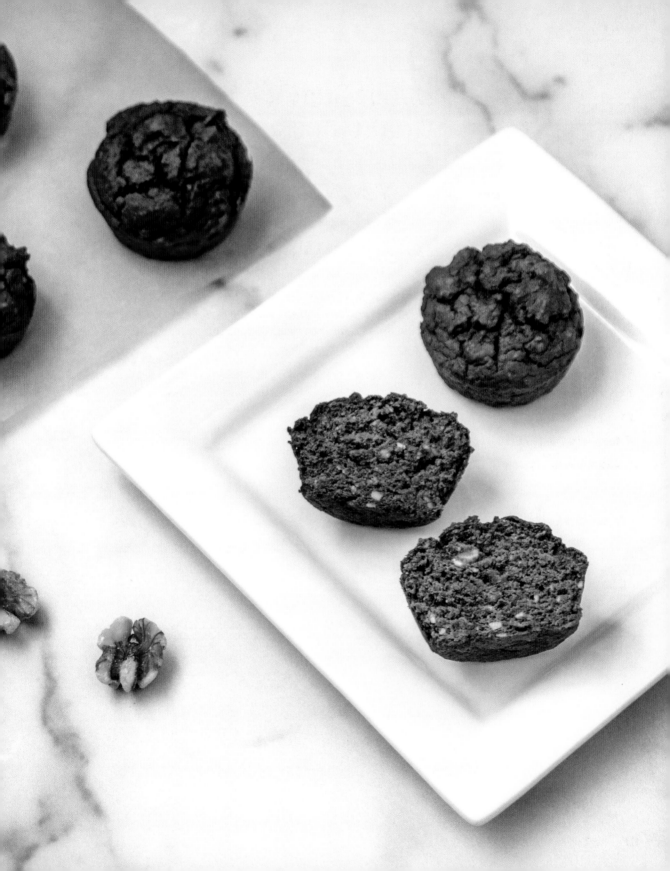

Beet Salad with Goat Cheese and SPICED WALNUTS

YIELD: 2 servings
PREP TIME: 5 minutes
COOK TIME: —

4 cups arugula

1 cup cooked and diced beets √

8 ounces extra-firm tofu, cubed and baked √

½ cup toasted and spiced walnuts √

2 ounces goat cheese, crumbled (optional)

¼ cup extra-virgin olive oil

1 tablespoon lemon juice

2 teaspoons Dijon mustard

1 teaspoon maple syrup

Salt and pepper

1. Divide the arugula evenly between two serving bowls.

2. Add the beets, tofu, spiced walnuts, and goat cheese, if using, to the bowls.

3. Make the dressing: In a small bowl, whisk together the oil, lemon juice, mustard, and maple syrup. Season with salt and pepper to taste. Use immediately, or store in the refrigerator for use later in the week.

4. Just before serving, drizzle the dressing over the salads.

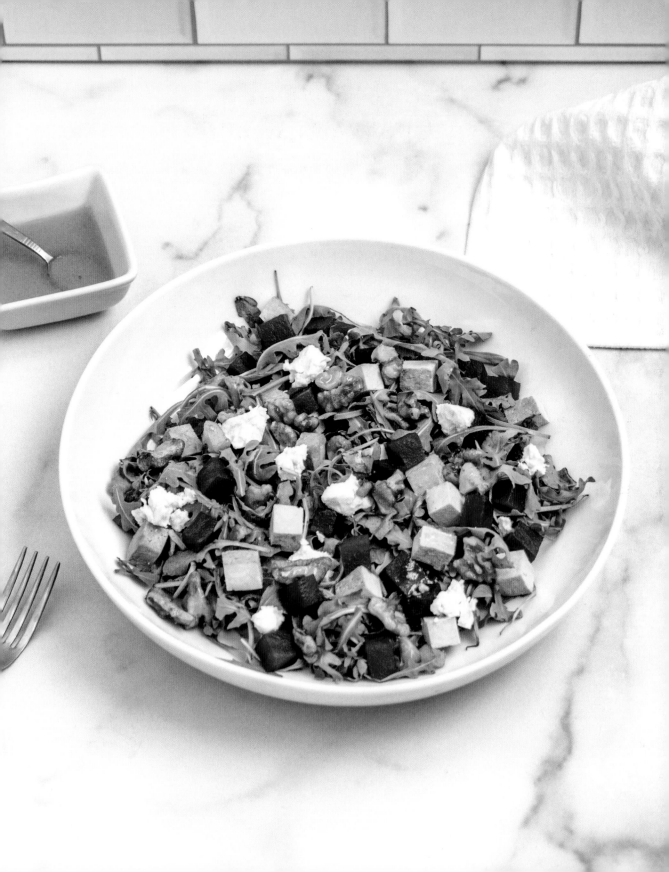

High-Protein
BLACK BEAN SOUP

YIELD: 2 servings
PREP TIME: 5 minutes
COOK TIME: 15 minutes

½ cup diced yellow onions √

1 tablespoon extra-virgin olive oil

2 cloves garlic, minced √

1 cup diced red bell peppers √

2 cups bone broth (chicken or beef)

1½ cups cooked black beans √

8 ounces extra-firm tofu, cubed

1 tablespoon lime juice

1 teaspoon chili powder

Salt and pepper

Fresh cilantro leaves, for garnish (optional)

NOTE:
This soup freezes well, so you can freeze any that you don't plan on eating within the week.

1. In a large saucepan over medium-high heat, sauté the onions in the oil until soft, about 3 minutes.

2. Add the garlic and bell peppers. Cook, stirring, for 3 more minutes.

3. Add the bone broth, beans, tofu, lime juice, and chili powder. Cover the pan and lower the heat to a simmer. Cook until the soup is heated through, about 10 minutes. Season with salt and pepper to taste.

4. Use a regular blender or an immersion blender to puree the soup, if desired. Serve garnished with cilantro, if desired, or store in the refrigerator for later in the week.

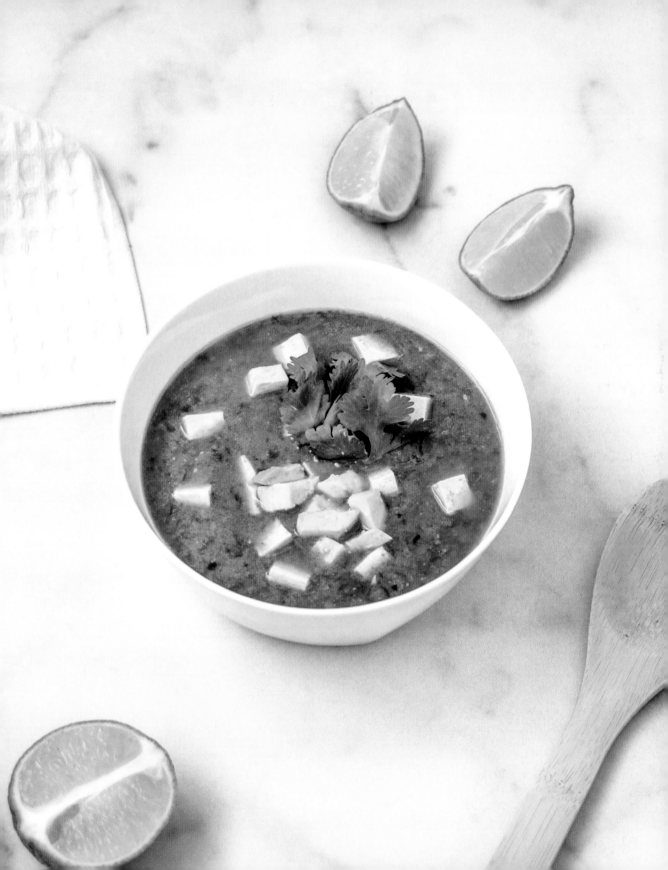

YIELD: 2 servings
PREP TIME: 10 minutes
COOK TIME: 30 minutes

Black Bean
ENCHILADAS

½ cup diced yellow onions √

½ cup diced green bell peppers √

2 tablespoons extra-virgin olive oil

8 ounces extra-firm tofu, cubed

4 cups fresh spinach, chopped √

1 cup cooked black beans √

1 teaspoon chili powder

Salt and pepper

4 low-carb whole-grain tortillas

2 cups prepared salsa √

¼ cup shredded Mexican blend cheese (optional)

Chopped fresh cilantro, for garnish (optional)

1. Preheat the oven to 400°F. Spray an 8-inch square baking dish with cooking spray.

2. In a large skillet over medium-high heat, sauté the onions and bell peppers in the oil until soft, about 3 minutes.

3. Add the tofu and cook, stirring, until it is starting to brown.

4. Add the spinach, beans, and chili powder to the pan and cook until the spinach is wilted and the beans are warmed through. Season with salt and pepper to taste.

5. Assemble the enchiladas: Fill each tortilla with one-quarter of the filling, roll tightly, and place seam side down in the prepared baking dish. Pour the salsa over the enchiladas and sprinkle with the cheese, if using.

6. Bake for 20 minutes, until golden. Serve garnished with cilantro, if desired, or store in the refrigerator for later in the week.

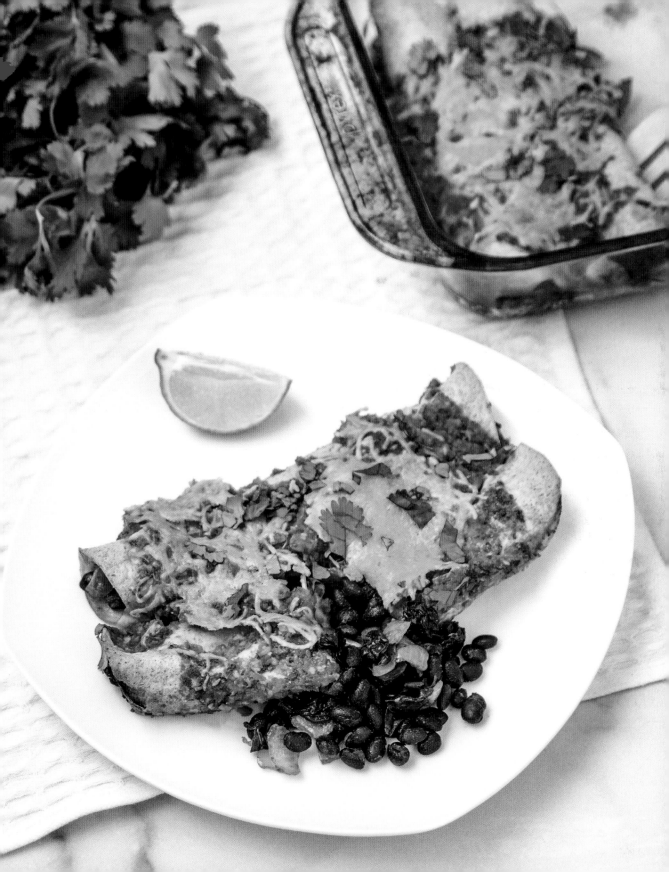

Black Bean Beet Burgers
with ROASTED
SPRING VEGGIES

YIELD: 2 servings
PREP TIME: 5 minutes
COOK TIME: 10 minutes

½ cup cooked black beans √

½ cup cooked and diced beets √

¼ cup diced yellow onions √

2 cloves garlic, minced, divided √

1 large egg

½ cup chickpea flour

¼ cup raw walnuts

¼ teaspoon fine sea salt

1 bundle asparagus, trimmed and chopped into 1-inch pieces √

1 cup sliced shiitake mushrooms √

2 tablespoons extra-virgin olive oil

Ground black pepper

1. Preheat the oven to 375°F. Line a sheet pan with parchment paper.

2. Put the beans, beets, onions, half of the minced garlic, the egg, chickpea flour, walnuts, and salt in a food processor and pulse until combined.

3. Form the mixture into 2 large patties, about 3 inches in diameter and 1½ inches thick, and place on the prepared pan. Bake for 20 minutes, carefully flipping the burgers over halfway through baking, until golden brown.

4. Meanwhile, place the asparagus, mushrooms, and remaining half of the minced garlic on a separate sheet pan. Drizzle with the oil and season with salt and pepper.

5. After the burgers have been in the oven for 5 minutes, put the pan with the veggies in the oven and bake them together for 15 minutes, until the vegetables are golden brown and the burgers are cooked through.

6. Serve, or store in the refrigerator for later in the week.

NOTE:
These burgers freeze well, so you can freeze any that you don't plan on eating within the week.

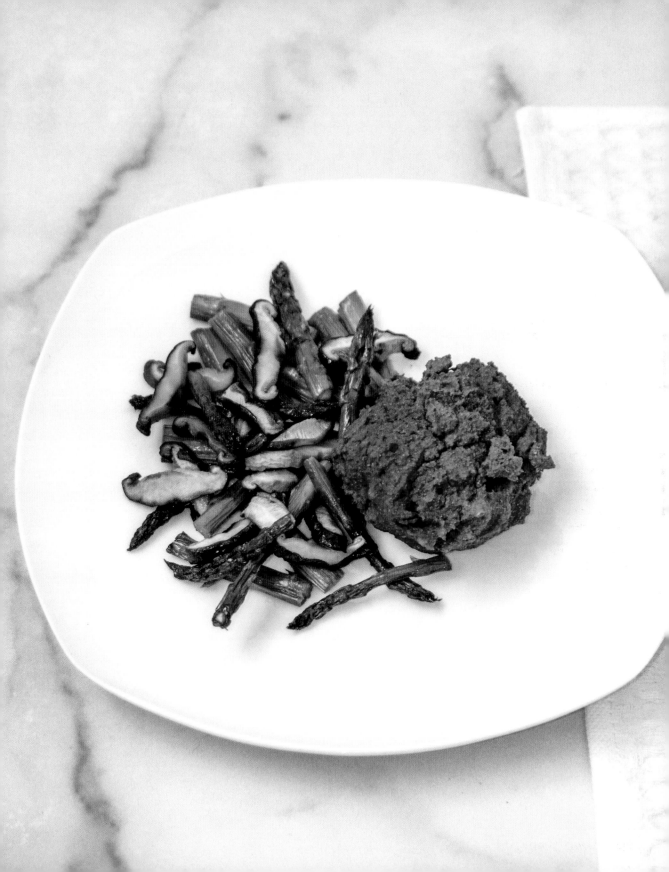

Week 7:

SHRIMP, OLIVE OIL, CHICKPEAS, AND PARSLEY

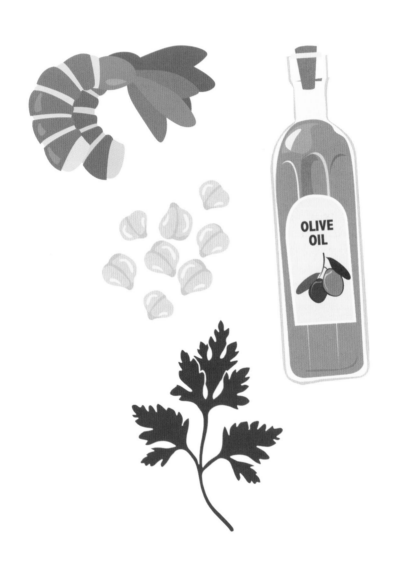

MENU

BREAKFAST	1	Greek Mini Quiches
	2	Spinach and Chickpea Egg Scramble
LUNCH	1	Cauliflower Tabbouleh with Chickpeas and Shrimp
	2	Chickpea and Spinach Shakshuka
DINNER	1	Spicy Shrimp and Broccoli with Spaghetti Squash
	2	Parsley Pesto Shrimp with Spaghetti Squash

FEATURED INGREDIENTS

 ### PROTEIN

This week's protein is shrimp, which is a lean protein source that is packed with omega-3 fatty acids. Omega-3 fatty acids are anti-inflammatory, and eating seafood at least twice per week has been linked to health benefits. Shrimp is also high in many beneficial nutrients for PCOS, including vitamin B12, zinc, and magnesium. You can buy fresh or frozen shrimp to use in this week's recipes.

 ### FIBER

Chickpeas are this week's main source of fiber. A half-cup of chickpeas contains more than 6 grams of fiber. They are also high in B vitamins, iron, magnesium, and zinc, making them a smart choice for PCOS. You can cook them from scratch, but they take a long time to cook, so it is more convenient to buy them in cans.

 ### FAT

This week's fat is olive oil, which is a staple of the anti-inflammatory Mediterranean diet. Extra-virgin olive oil adds a delicious flavor to almost any dish.

 ### PCOS POWER FOOD

This week's PCOS Power Food is fresh parsley, which is high in nutrients and antioxidants. More than just a culinary herb, this low-calorie leafy green has many benefits for health.

WEEKLY INGREDIENTS

FRESH PRODUCE

Baby kale, 1 cup

Broccoli, 1 small head

Cauliflower, 1 head (or 3 cups riced cauliflower)

Cherry tomatoes, 2 pints

Cucumber, 1

Garlic, 14 cloves

Green onions, 4

Parsley, curly or Italian, 3 cups (2 to 3 bunches)

Red bell peppers, 2

Spaghetti squash, 2 small

Spinach, 4 cups

Yellow onions, 3

MEAT/SEAFOOD

Shrimp (fresh or frozen), jumbo (16/20 size), 1¾ pounds

EGGS/DAIRY/MILK

Eggs, 20 large

Feta cheese, 4 ounces (optional, for quiches and egg scramble)

Parmesan cheese, grated, 2 tablespoons (optional)

Unsweetened nondairy milk of choice, ¼ cup

PANTRY

Cashews, ¼ cup

Chickpeas, 4 (15-ounce) cans

Diced tomatoes, 1 (28-ounce) can

Lemon juice, 3 tablespoons

Olive oil, extra-virgin, ¾ cup plus 1 tablespoon

Tomato paste, 2 tablespoons

SEASONINGS

Crushed red pepper, ½ teaspoon

Paprika, 2 teaspoons

CUSTOMIZING THE PLAN

TO ADD MORE CARBS:

- Have a piece of toast with the Greek Mini Quiches.
- Add bread or brown rice to the Shakshuka.
- Use brown rice in place of the cauliflower in the Cauliflower Tabbouleh.
- Replace the spaghetti squash with whole-grain pasta in the two dinner recipes.

TO MAKE THIS WEEK DAIRY-FREE:

- Omit the cheeses.

PREP DAY

Today you will be cooking the spaghetti squash, making the pesto, and prepping some of the vegetables for the week. Start with the squash since it takes the longest to cook. Also make the Greek Mini Quiches (page 132) so that they are ready to go in the mornings.

Complete the following tasks and store each component in a separate container in the refrigerator for use later in the week.

BAKE THE SQUASH

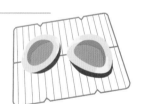

PREP TIME: 2 minutes
COOK TIME: 1 hour

Preheat the oven to 400°F.
Place 2 small spaghetti squash directly on the oven rack and bake for 1 hour. Remove from the oven and let cool. When cool enough to handle, cut each squash down the middle, scoop out and discard the seeds using a spoon, and then scrape out the "noodles" with a fork.

MAKE THE PARSLEY PESTO

YIELD: 1½ cups
PREP TIME: 5 minutes
COOK TIME: —

1 cup baby kale

1 cup fresh parsley

¼ cup cashews

¼ cup extra-virgin olive oil

2 cloves garlic, peeled

2 tablespoons grated Parmesan cheese (optional)

1 tablespoon lemon juice

¼ teaspoon fine sea salt

Put the ingredients in a food processor and pulse until well combined.

RICE THE CAULIFLOWER

Trim a head of cauliflower and cut it into chunks. Using a food processor, pulse until the cauliflower has the texture of rice. Store 3 cups in the refrigerator for use later in the week. (There may be extra, depending on the size of the head of cauliflower you purchased.)

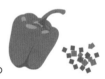

DICE THE YELLOW ONIONS

Dice enough yellow onions to measure 2½ cups.

SLICE THE GREEN ONIONS

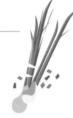

Thinly slice 4 green onions.

DICE THE PEPPER

Dice enough red bell pepper to measure 1 cup.

DICE THE CUCUMBER

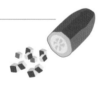

Dice enough cucumber to measure 1 cup.

CHOP THE SPINACH

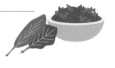

Roughly chop enough fresh spinach to measure 4 cups.

CHOP THE BROCCOLI

Chop enough broccoli into bite-sized pieces to measure 2 cups.

HALVE THE TOMATOES

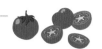

Halve enough cherry tomatoes to measure 3½ cups.

CHOP THE PARSLEY

Finely chop enough fresh parsley leaves to measure 2 cups.

MINCE THE GARLIC

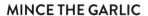
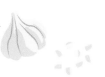

Mince 12 cloves of garlic.

YIELD: 8 mini quiches (2 per serving)
PREP TIME: 5 minutes
COOK TIME: 25 minutes

Greek
MINI QUICHES

4 ounces jumbo (16/20) shrimp (fresh or frozen), peeled and deveined

½ cup riced cauliflower √

½ cup halved cherry tomatoes √

¼ cup chopped fresh parsley √

2 ounces feta cheese, crumbled (optional)

6 large eggs

2 tablespoons unsweetened nondairy milk of choice

1 tablespoon extra-virgin olive oil

Salt and pepper

1. Preheat the oven to 350°F. Spray 8 wells of a standard-size muffin tin with cooking spray.

2. If using cooked frozen shrimp, defrost it under cold running water. If you purchased raw shrimp, bring a small pot of water to a boil. Add the shrimp and cook just until they turn pink, about 5 minutes. Drain and let cool. Coarsely chop the shrimp and set aside.

3. In a large bowl, combine the riced cauliflower, tomatoes, parsley, and feta, if using. Add the shrimp and stir to combine.

4. Divide the vegetable and shrimp mixture evenly among the greased wells of the muffin tin.

5. In a medium bowl, whisk the eggs, milk, and oil and season with salt and pepper.

6. Pour the egg mixture evenly over the vegetable and shrimp mixture in the muffin cups, filling them about two-thirds full.

7. Bake for 25 minutes, until the centers of the quiches are firm. Remove from the oven and let cool. Serve, or store in the refrigerator for later in the week.

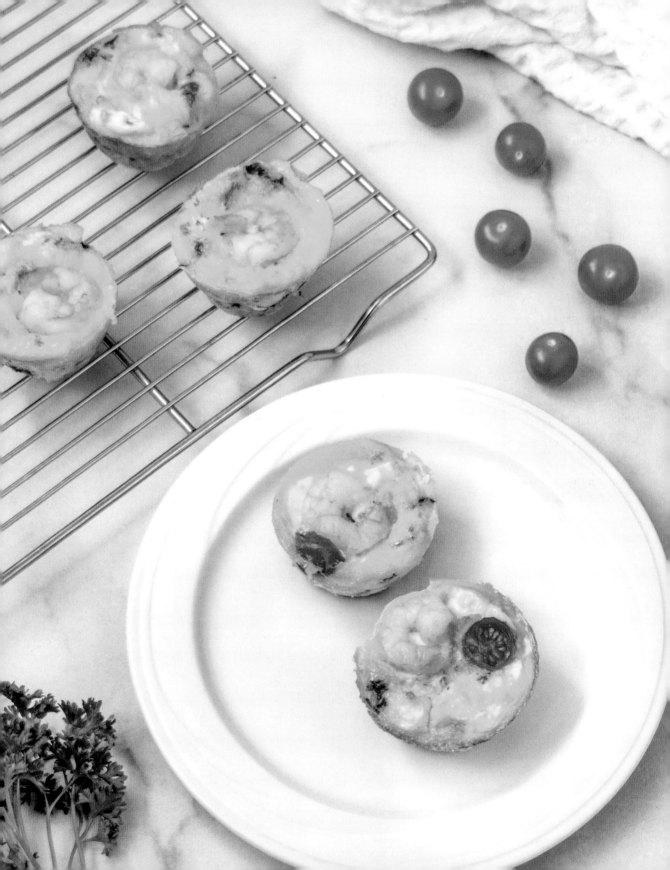

Spinach and Chickpea
EGG SCRAMBLE

YIELD: 2 servings
PREP TIME: 5 minutes
COOK TIME: 10 minutes

½ cup diced yellow onions √

1 tablespoon extra-virgin olive oil

4 large eggs

4 large egg whites

2 tablespoons unsweetened nondairy milk of choice

2 cloves garlic, minced √

2 cups chopped fresh spinach √

1 cup halved cherry tomatoes √

1 cup chickpeas, drained and rinsed

½ cup chopped fresh parsley √

2 ounces feta cheese, crumbled (optional)

Salt and pepper

1. In a large skillet over medium-high heat, sauté the onions in the oil until soft, about 3 minutes.

2. In a medium bowl, whisk the whole eggs, egg whites, and milk.

3. Pour the egg mixture into the pan with the onions and add the garlic, spinach, tomatoes, chickpeas, and parsley. Cook, stirring, until the eggs are set, about 5 minutes.

4. Add the feta, if using, and season with salt and pepper to taste.

5. Serve, or store in the refrigerator for later in the week.

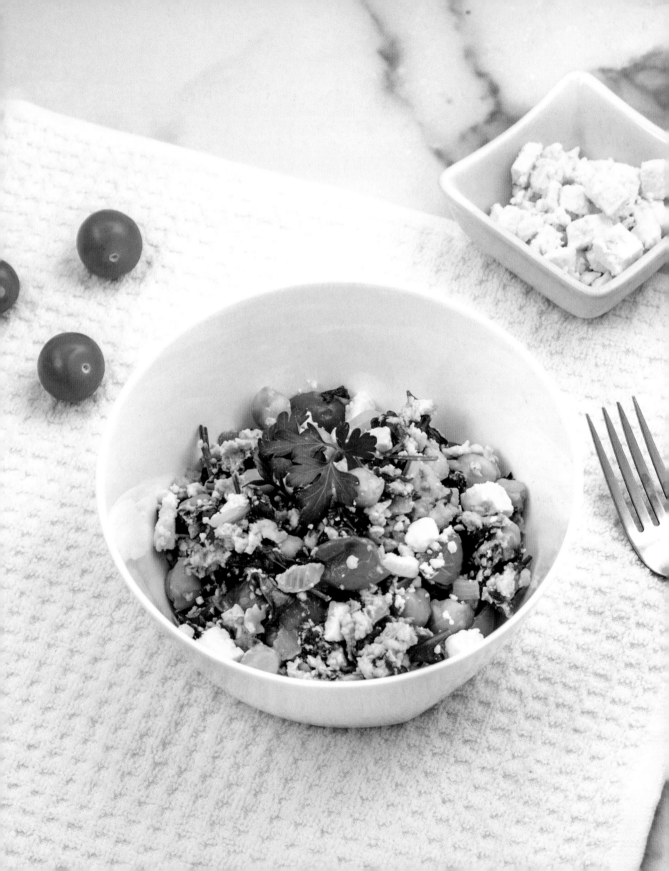

Cauliflower Tabbouleh
with CHICKPEAS and SHRIMP

YIELD: 2 servings
PREP TIME: 10 minutes
COOK TIME: —

8 ounces jumbo (16/20) shrimp (fresh or frozen), peeled and deveined

2 cups riced cauliflower √

1 cup halved cherry tomatoes √

1 cup diced cucumbers √

1 cup chopped fresh parsley √

4 green onions, sliced √

2 cloves garlic, minced √

1 (15-ounce) can chickpeas, drained and rinsed

2 tablespoons extra-virgin olive oil

2 tablespoons lemon juice

1 teaspoon paprika

¼ teaspoon fine sea salt

1. If using cooked frozen shrimp, defrost it under cold running water. If you purchased raw shrimp, bring a small pot of water to a boil. Add the shrimp and cook just until they turn pink, about 5 minutes. Drain and let cool. Coarsely chop the shrimp and set aside.

2. Make the tabbouleh: In a large bowl, combine the riced cauliflower, tomatoes, cucumbers, parsley, green onions, garlic, and chickpeas.

3. Make the dressing: Put the oil, lemon juice, paprika, and salt in a small jar and shake to combine. Pour the dressing over the tabbouleh and gently toss to combine.

4. Divide the tabbouleh between two plates and top with the shrimp.

5. Serve, or store in the refrigerator for later in the week.

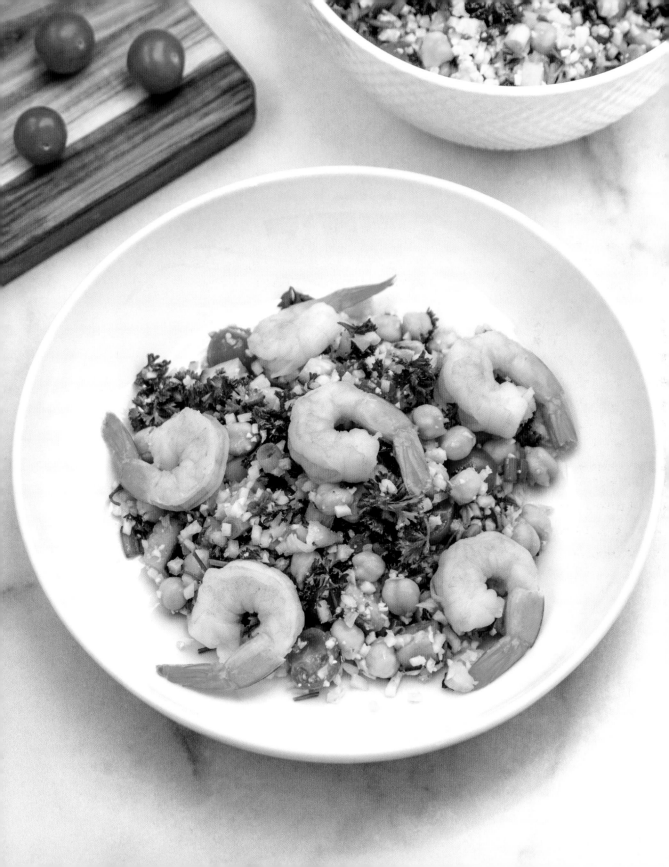

YIELD: 2 servings
PREP TIME: 5 minutes
COOK TIME: 20 minutes

Chickpea and Spinach
SHAKSHUKA

½ cup diced yellow onions √

2 tablespoons extra-virgin olive oil

1 (28-ounce) can diced tomatoes, with juice

2 tablespoons tomato paste

4 cloves garlic, minced √

1 teaspoon paprika

1 (15-ounce) can chickpeas, drained and rinsed

2 cups chopped fresh spinach √

6 large eggs

¼ teaspoon crushed red pepper

1. In a large skillet over medium-high heat, sauté the onions in the oil until soft.

2. Add the diced tomatoes with juice, tomato paste, garlic, and paprika and cook for 5 minutes.

3. Add the chickpeas and spinach and cook until the chickpeas are warmed through and the spinach is wilted, about 3 minutes.

4. Using a spoon, make 4 indentations in the sauce and crack an egg into each indent.

5. Reduce the heat to low and cover the skillet. Cook for 5 minutes, or until the eggs are set on top.

6. Sprinkle with the crushed red pepper and serve, or store in the refrigerator for later in the week.

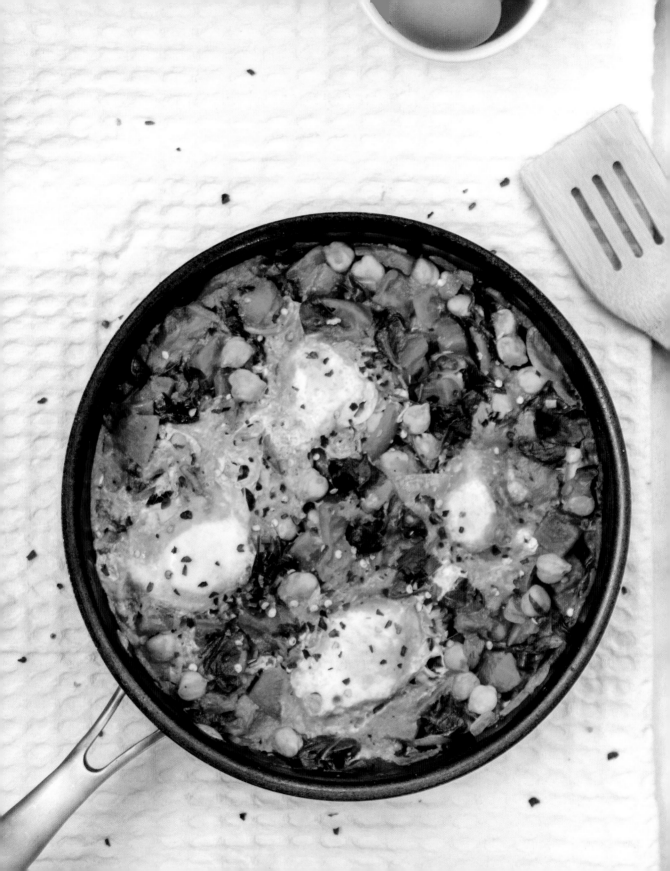

YIELD: 2 servings
PREP TIME: 5 minutes
COOK TIME: 20 minutes

Spicy Shrimp and Broccoli with
SPAGHETTI SQUASH

"Noodles" from 1 small spaghetti squash √

1 cup diced red bell peppers √

½ cup diced yellow onions √

2 tablespoons extra-virgin olive oil

2 cups chopped broccoli √

4 cloves garlic, minced √

8 ounces jumbo (16/20) shrimp (fresh or frozen), peeled and deveined

1 cup chickpeas, drained and rinsed

¼ cup chopped fresh parsley √

1 tablespoon lemon juice

¼ teaspoon crushed red pepper

1. Warm the spaghetti squash in the microwave or on the stovetop, then divide it evenly between two plates.

2. In a large skillet over medium-high heat, sauté the bell peppers and onions in the oil until soft, about 3 minutes.

3. Add the broccoli and garlic and cook, stirring, for 2 minutes, until the broccoli is crisp-tender.

4. Add the shrimp, chickpeas, parsley, lemon juice, and crushed red pepper. Cook just until the shrimp turn pink (or until warmed through if using cooked frozen shrimp), about 5 minutes.

5. Top the squash with the shrimp and broccoli mixture and serve, or store in the refrigerator for later in the week.

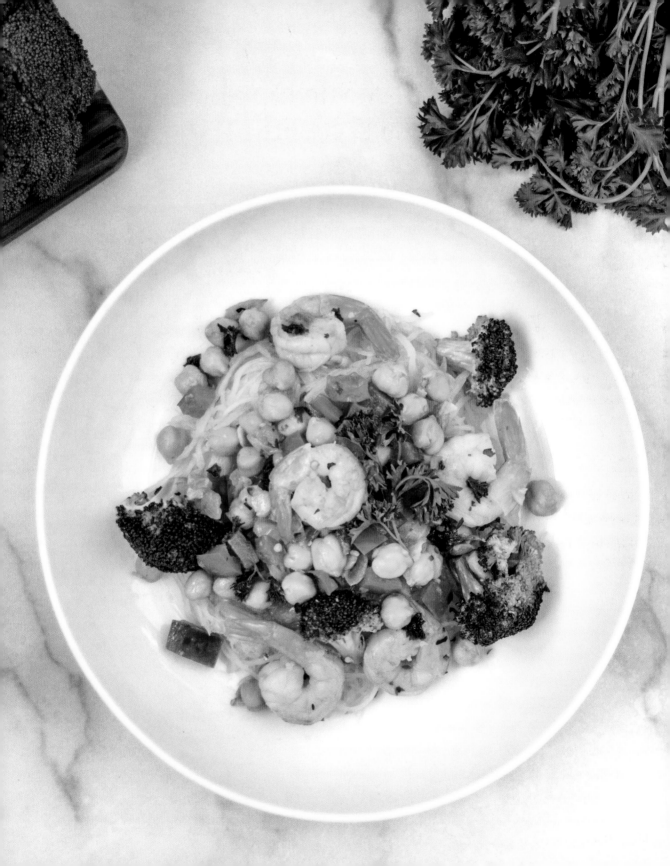

Parsley Pesto Shrimp
with SPAGHETTI SQUASH

YIELD: 2 servings
PREP TIME: 5 minutes
COOK TIME: about 10 minutes

"Noodles" from 1 small spaghetti squash √

8 ounces jumbo (16/20) shrimp (fresh or frozen), peeled and deveined

1 tablespoon extra-virgin olive oil

1 batch Parsley Pesto √

1 cup halved cherry tomatoes √

Salt and pepper

1. Warm the spaghetti squash in the microwave or on the stovetop, then divide it evenly between two plates.

2. In a large skillet over medium-high heat, sauté the shrimp in the oil just until it turns pink (or until warmed through if using frozen shrimp).

3. Stir in the pesto and tomatoes and season with salt and pepper to taste.

4. Top the squash with the shrimp and broccoli mixture and serve, or store in the refrigerator for later in the week.

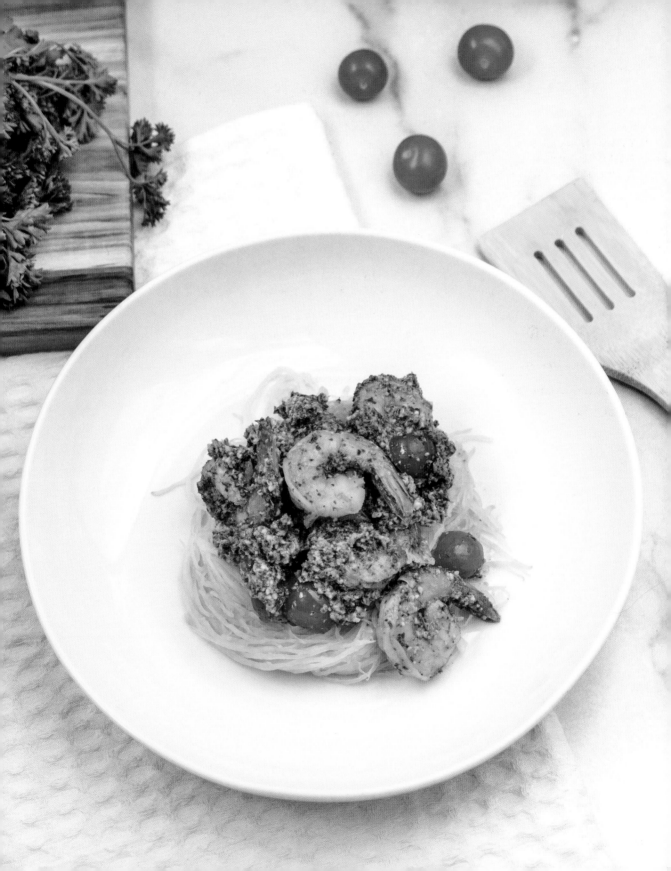

Week 8:

STEAK, AVOCADO OIL, ASPARAGUS, AND TURMERIC

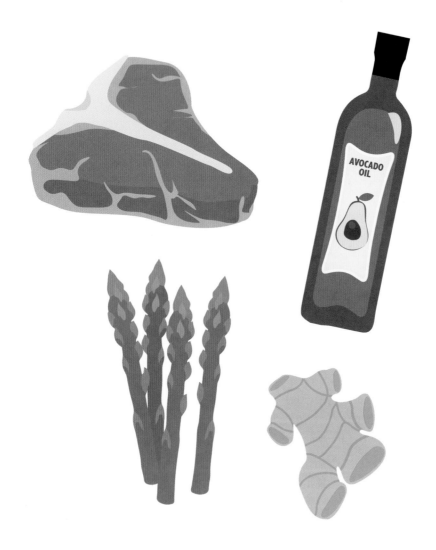

MENU

BREAKFAST	1	Anti-Inflammatory Asparagus Egg Scramble
	2	Turmeric Latte Chia Pudding
LUNCH	1	Turmeric Potato Salad
	2	Steak Salad with Asparagus and Potatoes
DINNER	1	One-Pan Steak and Potatoes
	2	Curried Beef Stew

FEATURED INGREDIENTS

PROTEIN

This week's protein is steak, which, depending on the cut you choose, can be a lean source of protein. Just 3 ounces of sirloin provides 26 grams of protein in 179 calories. Beef is a good source of nutrients important for PCOS, including vitamin B12 and zinc. Trim any visible fat off the steak before cooking.

FIBER

Asparagus is this week's main source of fiber. One cup contains nearly 3 grams of fiber and only 27 calories. Asparagus is also high in beta carotene, vitamin C, folate, and iron.

FAT

This week's fat is avocado oil, which is a neutral-tasting oil with a high smoke point, which means that it is safe to use for cooking at higher temperatures. Avocado oil is a good source of healthy monounsaturated fat.

PCOS POWER FOOD

This week's PCOS Power Food is turmeric powder, which contains curcumin, a potent natural anti-inflammatory. It is also high in beneficial plant compounds and antioxidants, making it especially beneficial for PCOS. Black pepper and fat increase the absorption and availability of curcumin in the bloodstream, so be sure to combine turmeric with black pepper and a source of fat for optimal effects.

WEEKLY INGREDIENTS

FRESH PRODUCE

Arugula, 8 cups

Asparagus, 2½ pounds

Button mushrooms, whole or sliced, 8 ounces

Carrots, 2

Cauliflower, 1 small head (or 1 cup riced cauliflower)

Cherry tomatoes, 1 pint

Garlic, 4 cloves

Green onions, 1 bunch

Kale, curly, 1 bunch

Parsley, curly or Italian, 1 bunch

Radishes, 4

Red potatoes, 2 pounds

Shallots, ½ cup

Yellow onion, 1

MEAT/SEAFOOD

Sirloin steak, boneless, 1½ pounds

EGGS/DAIRY/MILK

Eggs, 1 dozen large

Unsweetened nondairy milk of choice, 2 cups plus 2 tablespoons

PANTRY

All-purpose flour or gluten-free 1-to-1 flour, 1 tablespoon

Apple cider vinegar, 3 tablespoons

Avocado oil, ¾ cup plus 1 tablespoon

Beef bone broth, 2 cups

Chia seeds, ½ cup

Collagen peptides, ¼ cup (2 scoops)

Cooking spray (avocado or olive oil)

Dijon mustard, 2 tablespoons

Maple syrup, 2 teaspoons

Vanilla extract, 2 teaspoons

SEASONINGS

Ginger powder, 1 teaspoon

Ground cinnamon, ½ teaspoon

Turmeric powder, 1 tablespoon plus ½ teaspoon

CUSTOMIZING THE PLAN

TO ADD MORE CARBS:

- Have a piece of toast with the Anti-Inflammatory Egg Scramble.

- Add ¼ cup of old-fashioned oats to the Turmeric Latte Chia Pudding.

- Double the potatoes.

PREP DAY

Today you will be cooking the potatoes, eggs, and asparagus and prepping some of the vegetables for the week. Start with the potatoes since those take the longest to cook. Also make the Turmeric Latte Chia Pudding (page 152) so that it is ready to go in the mornings.

Complete the following tasks and store each component in a separate container in the refrigerator for use later in the week.

HALVE AND BOIL THE POTATOES

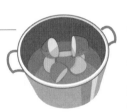

PREP TIME: 5 minutes
COOK TIME: 30 minutes

Halve 2 pounds red potatoes and place in a stockpot. Cover with water, add ½ teaspoon fine sea salt, and bring to a boil over medium-high heat. Cover and lower the heat to a simmer. Cook until tender, 25 to 30 minutes.

HARD-BOIL SOME OF THE EGGS

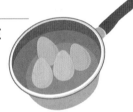

PREP TIME: 2 minutes
COOK TIME: 10 minutes

Put 4 eggs in a small saucepan and cover completely with water. Bring to a boil over medium-high heat. When the water reaches a boil, turn off the heat and let the eggs sit in the hot water for 10 minutes. Drain the hot water and fill the pan with cold water. When the eggs are cool, peel them.

CHOP AND STEAM THE ASPARAGUS

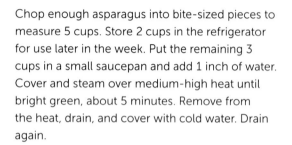

PREP TIME: 5 minutes
COOK TIME: 5 minutes

Chop enough asparagus into bite-sized pieces to measure 5 cups. Store 2 cups in the refrigerator for use later in the week. Put the remaining 3 cups in a small saucepan and add 1 inch of water. Cover and steam over medium-high heat until bright green, about 5 minutes. Remove from the heat, drain, and cover with cold water. Drain again.

RICE THE CAULIFLOWER

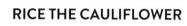

Trim a small head of cauliflower and cut it into chunks. Using a food processor, pulse until the cauliflower has the texture of rice. Store 1 cup in the refrigerator for use later in the week. (There may be extra, depending on the size of the head of cauliflower you purchased.)

DICE THE YELLOW ONION

Dice enough yellow onion to measure 1 cup.

SLICE THE GREEN ONIONS

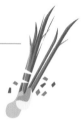

Thinly slice 6 green onions.

SLICE THE SHALLOTS

Thinly slice enough shallots to measure ½ cup.

SLICE THE RADISHES

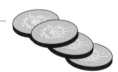

Thinly slice 4 radishes.

SLICE THE MUSHROOMS

Slice enough mushrooms to measure 2 cups. (If you bought presliced mushrooms, skip this step.)

CHOP THE CARROTS

Peel (if desired) and slice 2 carrots.

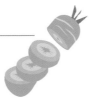

CHOP THE KALE

Roughly chop enough kale to measure 2 cups, removing any tough stems.

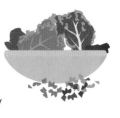

HALVE THE TOMATOES

Halve 1 pint of cherry tomatoes.

MINCE THE GARLIC

Mince 4 cloves of garlic.

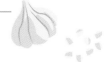

CHOP THE PARSLEY

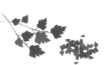

Finely chop enough fresh parsley leaves to measure ¼ cup.

Anti-Inflammatory Asparagus
EGG SCRAMBLE

YIELD: 2 servings
PREP TIME: 5 minutes
COOK TIME: 10 minutes

1 cup riced cauliflower √

2 tablespoons avocado oil

One-third of the steamed chopped asparagus √

2 green onions, thinly sliced √

4 large eggs

4 large egg whites

2 tablespoons unsweetened nondairy milk of choice

½ teaspoon turmeric powder

Salt and pepper

1. In a large skillet over medium-high heat, sauté the riced cauliflower in the oil until soft.

2. Add the asparagus and green onions and cook until heated through.

3. Meanwhile, in a medium bowl, whisk together the whole eggs, egg whites, milk, and turmeric.

4. Pour the egg mixture into the pan with the vegetables and cook, stirring, until the eggs are cooked through, about 5 minutes. Season with salt and pepper to taste.

5. Serve, or store in the refrigerator for later in the week.

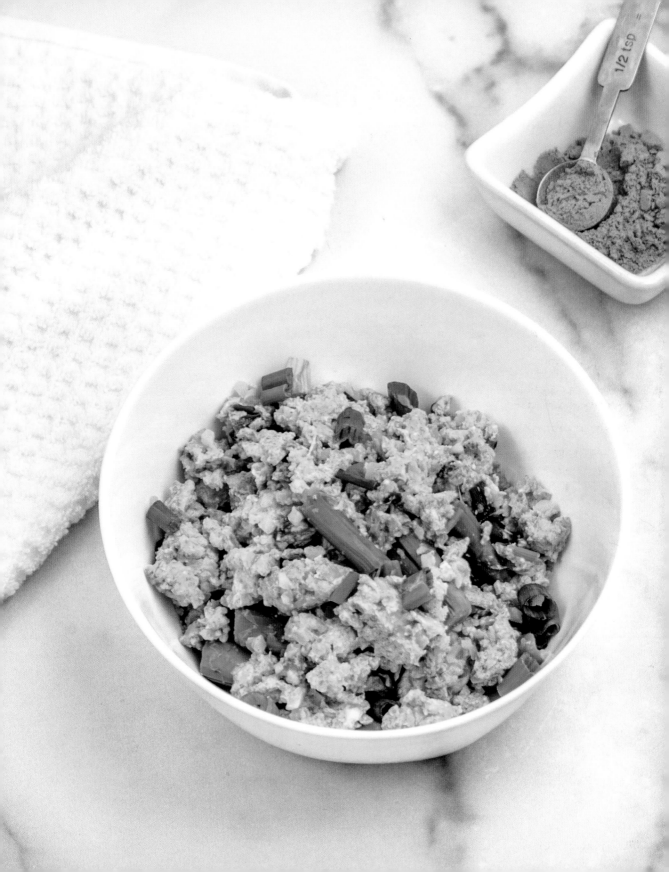

Turmeric Latte
CHIA PUDDING

YIELD: 2 servings
PREP TIME: 5 minutes
COOK TIME: 2 minutes

2 cups unsweetened nondairy milk of choice

2 teaspoons maple syrup

2 teaspoons vanilla extract

1 teaspoon turmeric powder

½ teaspoon ground cinnamon

⅛ teaspoon ground black pepper

½ cup chia seeds

¼ cup (2 scoops) collagen peptides

1. Heat the milk in a small saucepan over medium-high heat.

2. Stir in the maple syrup, vanilla, turmeric, cinnamon, and pepper. Remove from the heat.

3. Meanwhile, divide the chia seeds and collagen evenly between two containers (pint-size mason jars are perfect).

4. Pour the milk mixture evenly into the containers. Cover tightly and shake to combine.

5. Refrigerate the pudding at least overnight before serving, shaking occasionally.

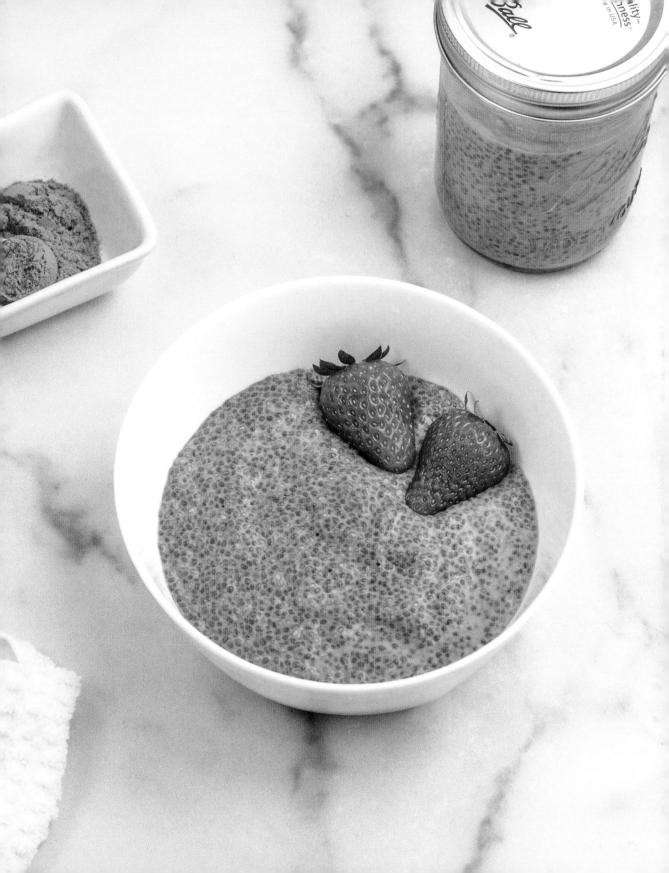

Turmeric
POTATO SALAD

YIELD: 2 servings
PREP TIME: 10 minutes
COOK TIME: —

One-quarter of the halved and boiled red potatoes √

4 hard-boiled eggs, peeled √

One-third of the steamed chopped asparagus √

4 green onions, thinly sliced √

2 tablespoons avocado oil

2 tablespoons apple cider vinegar

1 tablespoon Dijon mustard

½ teaspoon turmeric powder

½ teaspoon ginger powder

Salt and pepper

4 cups arugula

1. Roughly chop the potatoes and eggs and place them in a large bowl. Add the asparagus and green onions and toss to combine.

2. Make the dressing: In a small bowl, whisk together the oil, vinegar, mustard, turmeric, and ginger. Season with salt and pepper to taste.

3. Pour the dressing over the potato mixture and stir to combine. Serve, or store in the refrigerator for later in the week.

4. To serve, divide the arugula between two plates and top with the potato salad.

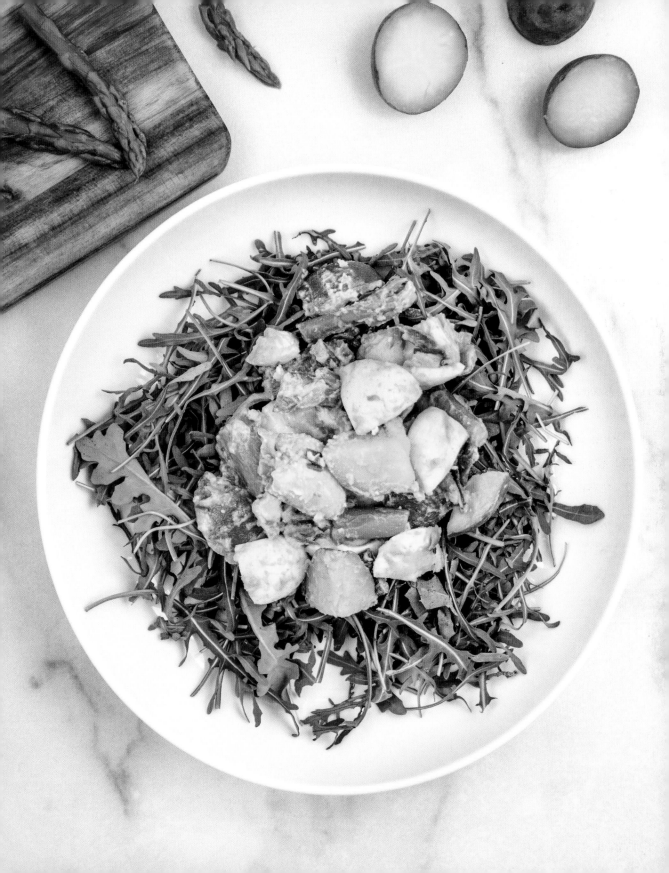

Steak Salad with
ASPARAGUS and
POTATOES

YIELD: 2 servings
PREP TIME: 10 minutes
COOK TIME: 10 minutes

8 ounces boneless sirloin steak

3 tablespoons avocado oil, divided

4 cups arugula

1 cup cherry tomatoes, halved √

4 radishes, thinly sliced √

One-third of the steamed chopped asparagus √

One-quarter of the halved and boiled red potatoes √

1 tablespoon apple cider vinegar

1 tablespoon Dijon mustard

½ teaspoon turmeric powder

Salt and pepper

1. In a large skillet over medium-high heat, cook the steak in 1 tablespoon of the oil for 3 to 4 minutes per side for medium doneness, or to the desired doneness. Remove from the pan and set aside.

2. Divide the arugula between two plates. Top with the tomatoes, radishes, asparagus, and potatoes.

3. Make the dressing: In a small bowl, whisk together the remaining 2 tablespoons of oil, the vinegar, mustard, and turmeric. Season with salt and pepper to taste.

4. When the steak is cool enough to handle, cut it into thin slices and top the salads with the steak. Drizzle the dressing over the salads and serve.

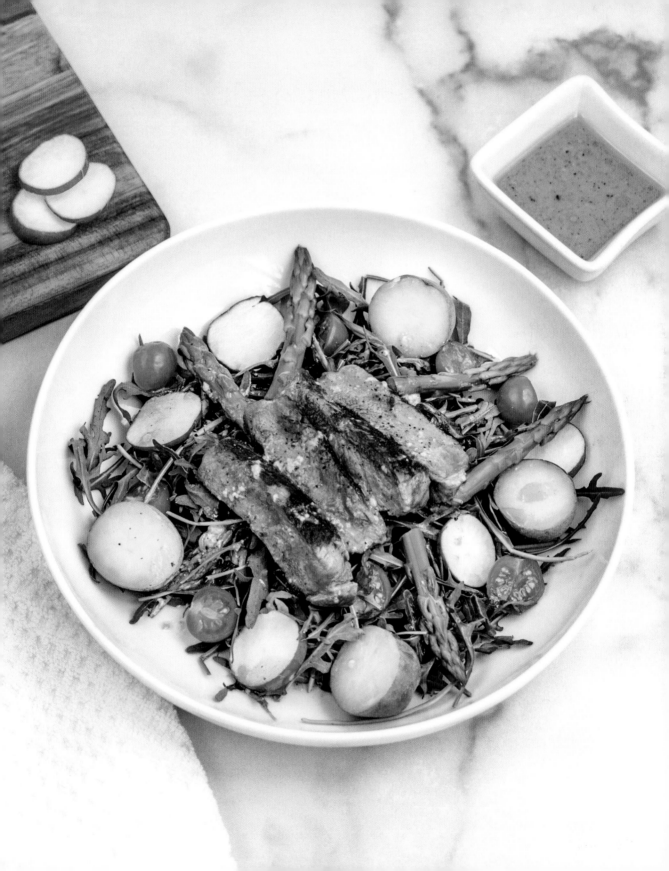

YIELD: 2 servings
PREP TIME: 5 minutes
COOK TIME: 25 minutes

One-Pan Steak and POTATOES

2 cups chopped asparagus √

2 cups sliced mushrooms √

One-quarter of the halved and boiled red potatoes √

1 cup cherry tomatoes, halved √

½ cup sliced shallots √

8 ounces boneless sirloin steak

2 tablespoons avocado oil

2 cloves garlic, minced √

¼ cup chopped fresh parsley √

Salt and pepper

1. Preheat the oven to 400°F and spray a sheet pan with cooking spray.

2. Place the asparagus, mushrooms, potatoes, tomatoes, and shallots on the prepared pan. Cut the steak into 1-inch pieces and add them to the pan.

3. Distribute the oil, garlic, and parsley over the ingredients on the pan and season everything with salt and pepper.

4. Bake for 25 minutes, until the steak is cooked to medium doneness and the vegetables are starting to brown. Remove from the oven and serve, or store in the refrigerator for later in the week.

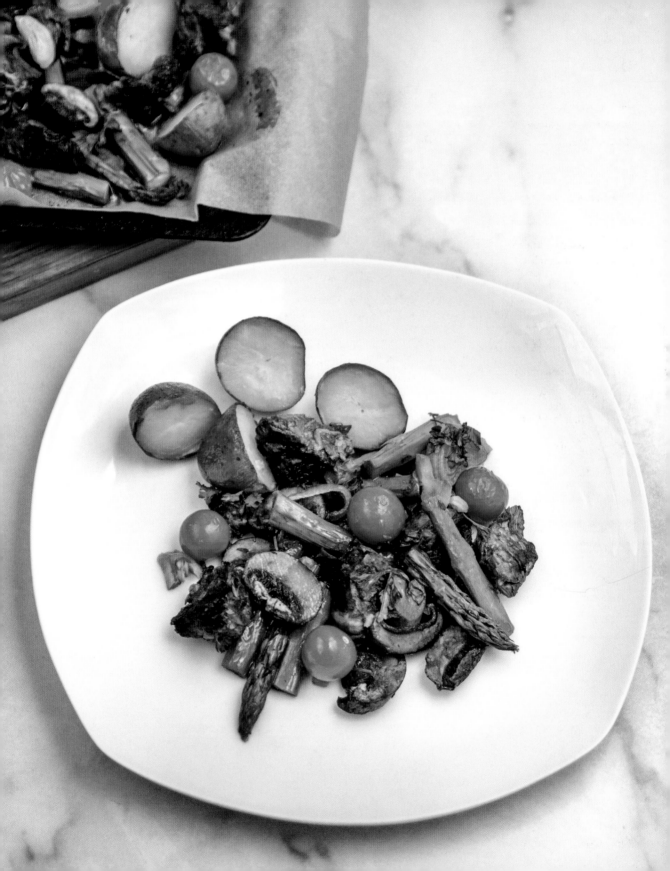

YIELD: 2 servings
PREP TIME: 5 minutes
COOK TIME: 20 minutes

Curried
BEEF STEW

8 ounces boneless sirloin steak, cut into 1-inch pieces

2 tablespoons avocado oil

2 carrots, chopped √

1 cup diced yellow onions √

One-quarter of the halved and boiled red potatoes √

2 cloves garlic, minced √

2 cups beef bone broth, divided

1 teaspoon turmeric powder

½ teaspoon ginger powder

2 cups chopped curly kale √

1 tablespoon all-purpose or gluten-free 1-to-1 flour

Salt and pepper

1. In a stockpot over medium-high heat, cook the steak in the oil until lightly browned on all sides, about 5 minutes.

2. Add the carrots, onions, potatoes, and garlic and cook, stirring often, until the onions have softened, about 5 minutes.

3. Add 1¾ cups of the broth, the turmeric, and ginger and cover the pot. Lower the heat and simmer for 5 minutes.

4. Add the kale and cook until softened, about 3 minutes.

5. Meanwhile, whisk the flour into the remaining ¼ cup of broth to make a slurry. Add the slurry to the pot and cook until the stew has thickened. Serve, or store in the refrigerator for later in the week.

NOTE:
This stew freezes well, so you can freeze any that you don't plan on eating within the week.

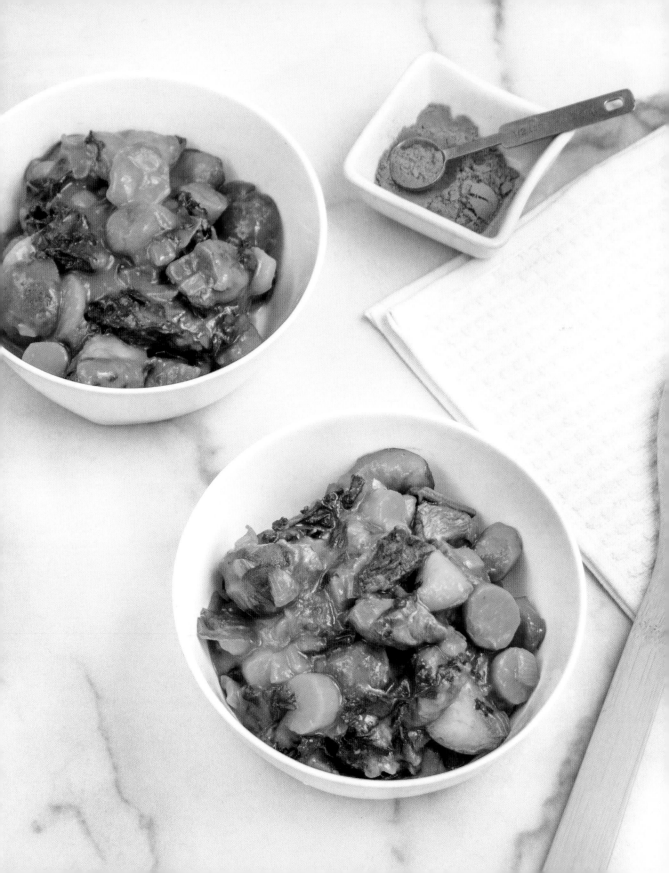

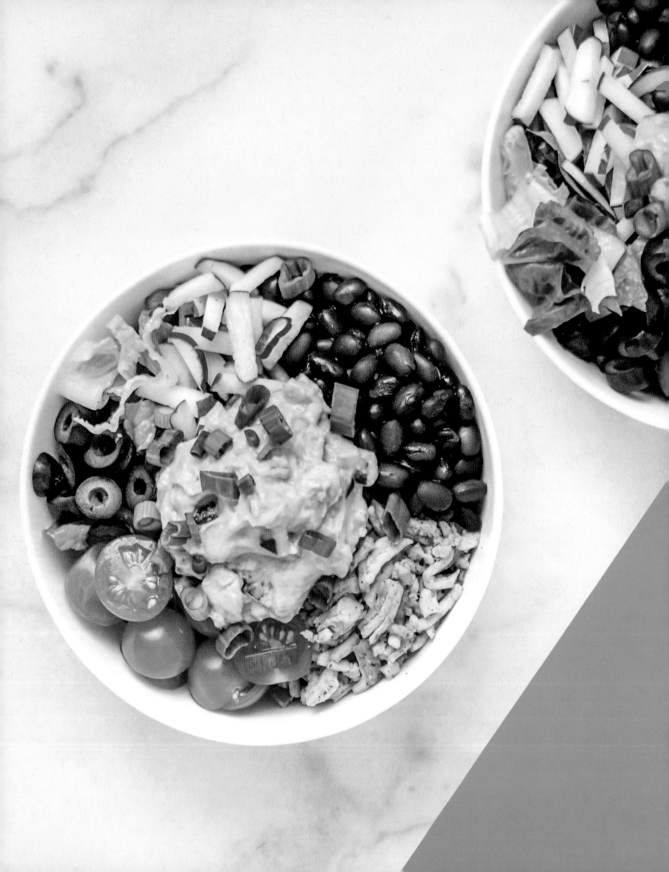

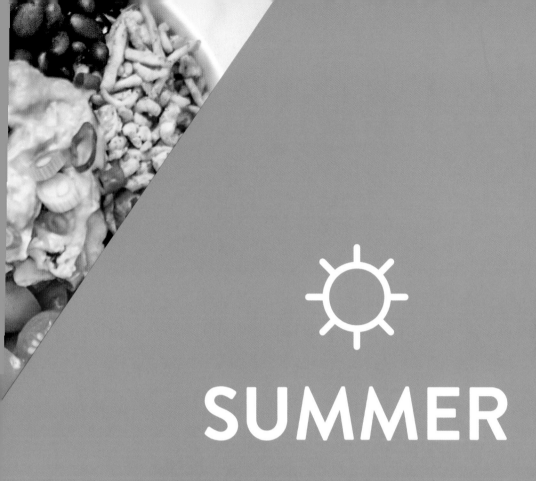

SUMMER

Week 9:

GROUND TURKEY, AVOCADO, RASPBERRIES, AND CHIA SEEDS

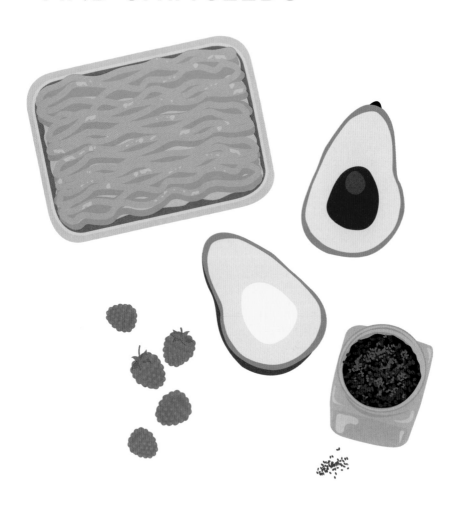

MENU

BREAKFAST	1	Raspberry Chocolate Chia Pudding
	2	Lemon-Berry Chia Muffins
LUNCH	1	Taco Lettuce Wraps with Guacamole
	2	Stuffed Summer Squash Boats
DINNER	1	Turkey Taco Bowls with Guacamole
	2	One-Pan Southwest Turkey Quinoa

FEATURED INGREDIENTS

 PROTEIN

This week's protein is ground turkey, which is a lean source of protein. Four ounces of 93 percent lean ground turkey provides 22 grams of protein in 167 calories. Turkey is a good source of nutrients important for PCOS, including vitamins B6 and B12.

 FIBER

Raspberries are this week's main source of fiber. One cup of raspberries provides a whopping 8 grams of fiber with only 65 calories. Raspberries are also high in vitamin C and contain some magnesium and iron as well.

 FAT

This week's fat is avocado, which is not only a good source of monounsaturated fats but also high in fiber. Avocados brown quickly after cutting, so they should not be prepped in advance.

 PCOS POWER FOOD

This week's PCOS Power Food is chia seeds. A 1-ounce serving provides 11 grams of fiber, 4 grams of protein, and 5 grams of omega-3 fatty acids. Chia seeds are high in many minerals, including magnesium and calcium. They are absorbed better when they are soaked in liquid.

WEEKLY INGREDIENTS

FRESH PRODUCE

Avocados, Hass, 3

Cherry tomatoes, 1 pint

Garlic, 3 cloves

Green onions, 4

Jalapeño pepper, 1

Poblano or green bell pepper, 1

Radishes, 8

Raspberries, 1 pint

Red onion, 1

Romaine lettuce, 2 heads

Spinach, 2 cups

Yellow onion, 1

Yellow summer squash, 2 large

FROZEN FOODS

Corn, ½ cup

MEAT/SEAFOOD

Ground turkey, 2 pounds

EGGS/DAIRY/MILK

Eggs, 4 large

Mexican blend cheese, shredded,
4 ounces (optional, for lettuce wraps
and squash boats)

Unsweetened nondairy milk of choice,
2 cups

PANTRY

Almond flour, blanched, ½ cup

Baking powder, 1 teaspoon

Black beans, 2 (15-ounce) cans

Black olives, sliced, ½ cup

Cacao powder or cocoa powder,
2 tablespoons

Chia seeds, ½ cup plus 2 tablespoons

Coconut oil, ¼ cup

Cooking spray (avocado or olive oil)

Lemon juice, 2 tablespoons

Lime juice, ½ cup

Maple syrup, 3 tablespoons

Protein powder, unflavored or vanilla-
flavored, ½ cup (4 scoops)

Quinoa, 1 cup

Vanilla extract, 2 teaspoons

SEASONINGS

Chili powder, 2 tablespoons

Ground cinnamon, ½ teaspoon

CUSTOMIZING THE PLAN

TO ADD MORE CARBS:

- Add ¼ cup old-fashioned oats to the Raspberry Chocolate Chia Pudding.

- Double the quinoa.

- Use whole-wheat flour in place of the almond flour in the Lemon-Berry Chia Muffins.

- Use whole-grain tortillas in place of the lettuce in the Taco Lettuce Wraps.

- Add quinoa to the Turkey Taco Bowls.

TO MAKE THIS WEEK DAIRY-FREE:

- Omit the cheese.

PREP DAY

Today you will be cooking the quinoa and some of the turkey, making the guacamole, and prepping some of the vegetables for the week. Also bake the Lemon-Berry Chia Muffins (page 170) and prepare the Raspberry Chocolate Chia Pudding (page 169). Start with the muffins and quinoa since those take the longest to cook.

Complete the following tasks and store each component in a separate container in the refrigerator for use later in the week.

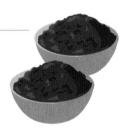

COOK THE QUINOA

YIELD: about 2 cups
PREP TIME: 5 minutes
COOK TIME: 20 minutes

In a medium saucepan over medium-high heat, combine 1 cup quinoa with 2 cups water and ¼ teaspoon fine sea salt. Bring to a boil, then cover, lower the heat to a simmer, and cook until all of the water is absorbed, about 20 minutes.

COOK AND SEASON SOME OF THE TURKEY

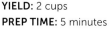

PREP TIME: 5 minutes
COOK TIME: 15 minutes

In a large skillet over medium-high heat, cook 1 pound of the ground turkey until it is no longer pink, breaking it up into smaller pieces. Add 1 tablespoon chili powder and season with salt and pepper to taste.

MAKE THE GUACAMOLE

YIELD: 2 cups
PREP TIME: 5 minutes
COOK TIME: —

In a large bowl, combine the flesh of 2 avocados, ¼ cup diced red onions, ½ diced jalapeño pepper, 2 tablespoons lime juice, and 1 clove minced garlic. Mash the avocado and stir to combine. Season with salt and pepper to taste.

MINCE THE GARLIC

Mince 3 cloves of garlic. Set one clove aside for the guacamole and store the rest for use later in the week.

DICE THE YELLOW ONIONS

Dice enough yellow onions to measure 1 cup.

DICE THE PEPPER

Dice 1 poblano or green bell pepper.

SLICE THE GREEN ONIONS

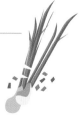

Thinly slice 4 green onions.

SLICE THE RADISHES

Thinly slice 8 radishes into matchsticks.

CHOP THE LETTUCE

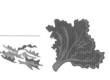

Chop enough romaine lettuce to measure 4 cups.

HALVE THE TOMATOES

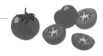

Halve 1 pint of cherry tomatoes.

Raspberry Chocolate
CHIA PUDDING

YIELD: 2 servings
PREP TIME: 5 minutes
COOK TIME: —

1. Heat the milk in a small saucepan over medium-high heat.

2. Stir in the cacao powder, maple syrup, vanilla, and cinnamon. Remove from the heat.

3. Meanwhile, divide the chia seeds and protein powder evenly between two containers (mason jars are perfect).

4. Pour the milk mixture evenly into the containers. Cover tightly and shake to combine.

5. Refrigerate the pudding at least overnight, shaking occasionally. Serve with the raspberries.

2 cups unsweetened nondairy milk of choice

2 tablespoons cacao powder or cocoa powder

2 teaspoons maple syrup

1 teaspoon vanilla extract

½ teaspoon ground cinnamon

½ cup chia seeds

¼ cup (2 scoops) unflavored or vanilla-flavored protein powder

1 cup fresh raspberries, for serving

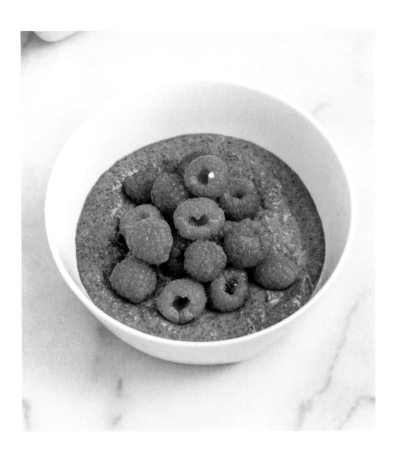

YIELD: 8 muffins (2 per serving)
PREP TIME: 5 minutes
COOK TIME: 25 minutes

Lemon-Berry
CHIA MUFFINS

½ cup blanched almond flour

¼ cup (2 scoops) unflavored or vanilla-flavored protein powder

2 tablespoons chia seeds

1 teaspoon baking powder

⅛ teaspoon fine sea salt

4 large eggs

¼ cup coconut oil, melted

2 tablespoons lemon juice

2 tablespoons maple syrup

1 teaspoon vanilla extract

1 cup fresh raspberries

1. Preheat the oven to 350°F and spray 8 wells of a standard-size muffin tin with cooking spray.

2. In a large bowl, whisk together the almond flour, protein powder, chia seeds, baking powder, and salt.

3. Add the eggs, coconut oil, lemon juice, maple syrup, and vanilla and stir to combine.

4. Roughly chop the raspberries and gently fold them into the batter.

5. Pour the batter evenly into the greased wells of the muffin tin, filling them two-thirds full. Bake for 22 to 25 minutes, until a toothpick inserted in the center of a muffin comes out clean.

6. Remove from the oven, transfer the muffins to a cooling rack, and let cool. Serve, or store for later in the week.

NOTE:
These muffins freeze well, so you can freeze any that you don't plan on eating within the week.

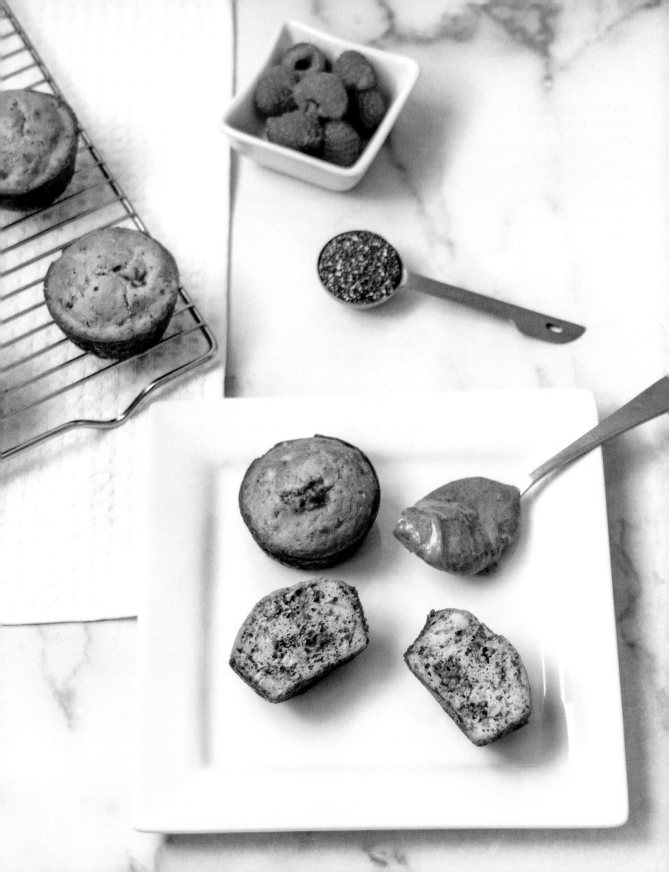

Taco Lettuce Wraps
with GUACAMOLE

YIELD: 2 servings
PREP TIME: 5 minutes
COOK TIME: —

4 romaine lettuce leaves

Half of the cooked and seasoned ground turkey √

1 cup guacamole √

2 ounces shredded Mexican blend cheese (optional)

4 radishes, sliced √

¼ cup sliced black olives

2 green onions, thinly sliced √

1. Place two lettuce leaves on each of two plates. Divide the turkey evenly among the leaves.

2. Top with the guacamole, cheese (if using), radishes, olives, and green onions and serve.

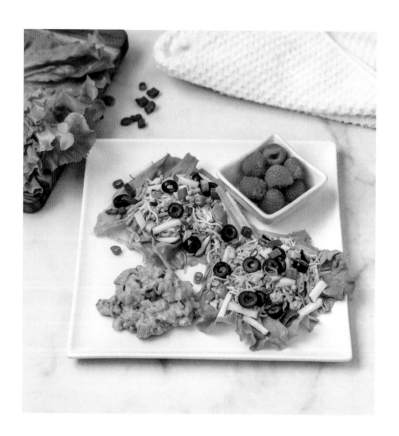

Stuffed Summer
SQUASH BOATS

YIELD: 2 servings
PREP TIME: 5 minutes
COOK TIME: 20 minutes

1. Preheat the oven to 350°F and spray a sheet pan with cooking spray or line it with parchment paper.

2. Slice the squash in half lengthwise and use a spoon to scoop out the seeds. Place the squash halves cut side up on the prepared sheet pan.

3. Stuff the squash halves with equal amounts of the turkey quinoa mixture and top with the cheese, if using. Season with salt and pepper to taste.

4. Bake for 20 minutes, or until lightly browned on top.

5. Serve, or store in the refrigerator for later in the week.

2 large yellow summer squash

½ recipe One-Pan Southwest Turkey Quinoa (page 176)

2 ounces shredded Mexican blend cheese (optional)

Salt and pepper

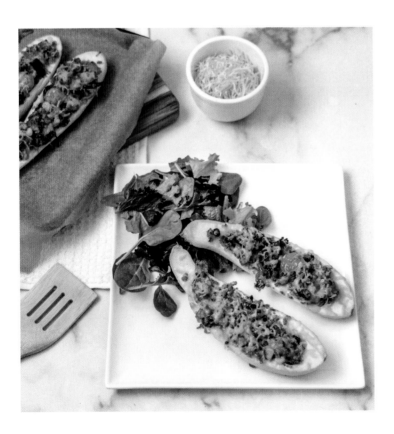

YIELD: 2 servings
PREP TIME: 10 minutes
COOK TIME: —

Turkey Taco Bowls
with GUACAMOLE

4 cups chopped romaine lettuce √

Half of the cooked and seasoned ground turkey √

1 cup canned black beans, drained and rinsed

4 radishes, sliced √

¼ cup sliced black olives

1 cup cherry tomatoes, halved √

1 cup guacamole √

2 green onions, thinly sliced √

1. Divide the lettuce evenly between two serving bowls.

2. Arrange the turkey, beans, radishes, olives, and tomatoes around the bowls. Top with the guacamole, sprinkle with the green onions, and serve.

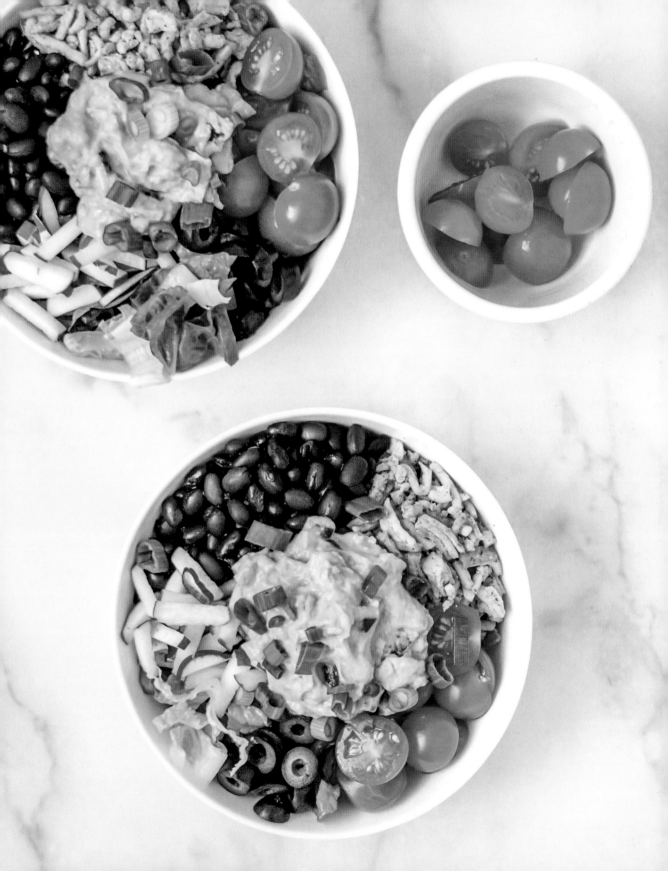

YIELD: 2 servings + 2 leftover servings for Spaghetti Squash Boats
PREP TIME: 5 minutes
COOK TIME: 20 minutes

One-Pan Southwest
TURKEY QUINOA

1 cup diced yellow onions √

2 tablespoons avocado oil

1 pound ground turkey

2 cloves garlic, minced √

1 poblano or green bell pepper, diced √

½ cup frozen corn

1 tablespoon chili powder

2 cups cooked quinoa √

1 cup canned black beans, drained and rinsed

2 cups fresh spinach

1 cup cherry tomatoes, halved √

Salt and pepper

1. In a large skillet over medium-high heat, sauté the onions in the oil until softened.

2. Add the turkey and cook, breaking up the meat into small pieces, until no longer pink, about 5 minutes.

3. Add the garlic, poblano pepper, corn, and chili powder and cook until the pepper is soft and the corn is no longer frozen, about 5 minutes.

4. Add the quinoa and black beans and cook until warmed through, about 5 minutes.

5. Add the spinach and tomatoes and cook until the spinach is wilted, about 5 minutes. Season with salt and pepper to taste.

6. Store half of the mixture in the refrigerator for use in the Stuffed Summer Squash Boats (page 173). Serve the remainder, or store in the refrigerator for later in the week.

NOTE:
This dish freezes well, so you can freeze any that you don't plan on eating within the week.

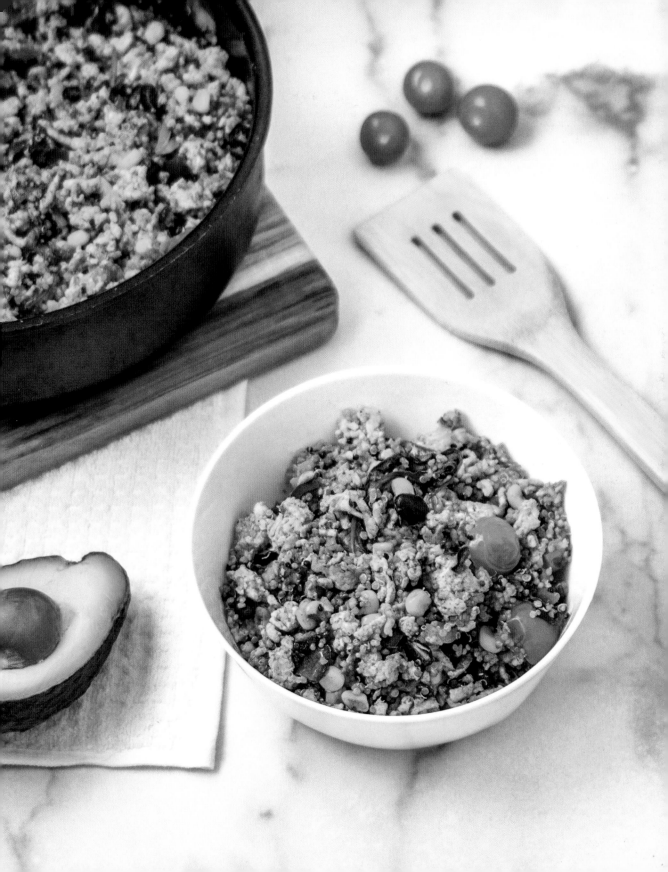

Week 10:

SALMON, PUMPKIN SEEDS, STRAWBERRIES, AND SPEARMINT

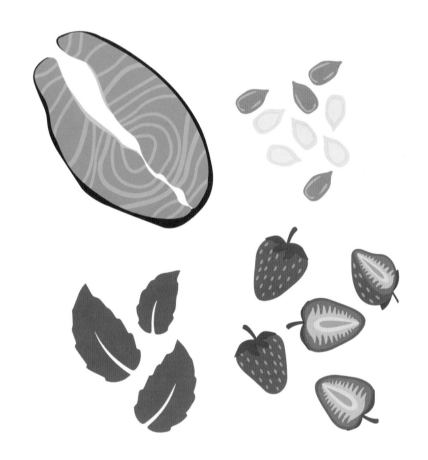

MENU

BREAKFAST	1	Summer Berry Parfaits
	2	Overnight Protein Oats with Strawberry Chia Jam
LUNCH	1	Deconstructed Summer Roll Salad
	2	Summer Salmon Salad
DINNER	1	Salmon with Pineapple-Mint Salsa
	2	Pumpkin-Crusted Salmon Sheet Pan Dinner

FEATURED INGREDIENTS

PROTEIN

This week's protein is salmon, which is especially beneficial for PCOS due to its high omega-3 fatty acid content. Omega-3s are anti-inflammatory, and eating seafood at least twice per week has been linked to health benefits. Ideally, you want to select wild-caught salmon, as it is higher in omega-3s than farm-raised salmon. If you can't find fresh salmon locally, frozen is fine; just remember to thaw it in the refrigerator before cooking.

FAT

This week's fat is pumpkin seeds, which are a good source of healthy polyunsaturated fats, protein, and fiber but also are high in nutrients important for PCOS, such as zinc and magnesium. Look for shelled green pumpkin seeds, also called pepitas.

FIBER

Strawberries are this week's main source of fiber. One cup of strawberries provides 3 grams of fiber and has only 47 calories. Strawberries are extremely high in vitamin C and low in sugar.

PCOS POWER FOOD

This week's PCOS Power Food is spearmint. Studies have shown that spearmint may help reduce androgens in women with PCOS and help with some androgen-driven symptoms, such as facial hair and hair loss. Spearmint is low in calories and adds a fresh, distinctive taste to many dishes. It can also be consumed as a tea.

WEEKLY INGREDIENTS

FRESH PRODUCE

Avocados, Hass, 2

Basil, ¼ cup

Blueberries, ½ cup

Broccolini, 2 cups

Carrot, 1

Cherry tomatoes, 1 cup

Cucumbers, 2

Garlic, 2 cloves

Green onions, 6

Mint, 1 bunch

Mixed greens, 10 cups

Pineapple, 1

Radishes, 8

Raspberries, ½ cup

Red cabbage, 1 cup shredded

Red onion, 1

Red potatoes, 1 cup

Strawberries, 2 pints

Tomatoes, 1 cup

MEAT/SEAFOOD

Salmon fillets, 8 (4 ounces each)

EGGS/DAIRY/MILK

Goat cheese, 2 ounces (optional)

Greek yogurt, full-fat plain, 2 cups

Unsweetened nondairy milk of choice, 1 cup

PANTRY

Avocado oil, ¼ cup

Balsamic glaze, 2 teaspoons

Black beans, 1 (15-ounce) can

Brown rice noodles, 4 ounces

Chia seeds, 1 tablespoon

Cooking spray (avocado or olive oil)

Ground flaxseed, 6 tablespoons

Lemon juice, 1 tablespoon

Lime juice, 3 tablespoons

Old-fashioned oats, ¾ cup

Protein powder, unflavored or vanilla-flavored, ½ cup (4 scoops)

Pumpkin seeds (pepitas), 1½ cups

Rice vinegar, 1 tablespoon

SEASONINGS

Ginger powder, ½ teaspoon

Ground cinnamon, 1 teaspoon

CUSTOMIZING THE PLAN

TO ADD MORE CARBS:

- Double the oats.

- Double the rice noodles.

- Double the black beans.

- Have a piece of toast with the Summer Berry Parfait.

TO MAKE THIS WEEK DAIRY-FREE:

- Omit the goat cheese.

- Use a nondairy yogurt in place of the Greek yogurt, but add protein powder to increase the protein content.

PREP DAY

Today you will be cooking the rice noodles and some of the salmon, making the pineapple salsa, and prepping some of the fruits and vegetables for the week. Also make the Summer Berry Parfaits (page 183) and the Overnight Protein Oats with Strawberry Chia Jam (page 184).

Complete the following tasks and store each component in a separate container in the refrigerator for use later in the week.

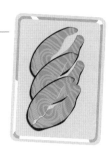

COOK THE RICE NOODLES

YIELD: 1 cup
PREP TIME: 5 minutes
COOK TIME: 10 minutes

Bring 4 cups water to a boil in a medium saucepan over medium-high heat. Add 4 ounces brown rice noodles and cook for 5 minutes. Drain and rinse.

BAKE SOME OF THE SALMON

PREP TIME: 2 minutes
COOK TIME: 20 minutes

Preheat the oven to 375°F. Line a sheet pan with parchment paper or spray it with cooking spray. Place 1 pound salmon fillets on the prepared pan, drizzle with 1 tablespoon lemon juice, and season with salt and pepper. Bake for 20 minutes, or until the salmon is opaque in the center.

CHOP THE MINT

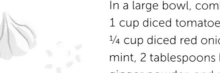

Chop enough mint to measure 1 cup. Set aside ¼ cup for the salsa and store the rest for use later in the week.

MAKE THE PINEAPPLE-MINT SALSA

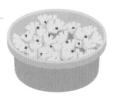

YIELD: 4 cups
PREP TIME: 10 minutes
COOK TIME: —

In a large bowl, combine 2 cups diced pineapple, 1 cup diced tomatoes, ½ cup diced cucumbers, ¼ cup diced red onions, ¼ cup chopped fresh mint, 2 tablespoons lime juice, ½ teaspoon ginger powder, and salt and pepper to taste. Stir to combine.

MINCE THE GARLIC

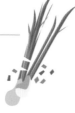

Mince 2 cloves of garlic.

SLICE THE GREEN ONIONS

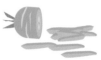

Thinly slice 6 green onions.

SLICE THE RADISHES

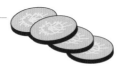

Thinly slice 8 radishes.

JULIENNE THE CARROT

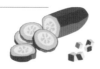

Peel and julienne a carrot into matchsticks.

SLICE SOME OF THE STRAWBERRIES

Slice 1 pint of strawberries.

SLICE THE CUCUMBER

Slice enough cucumber to measure 1 cup.

SHRED THE CABBAGE

Shred enough red cabbage to measure 1 cup. (If you bought preshredded cabbage, skip this step.)

Summer
BERRY PARFAITS

YIELD: 2 servings
PREP TIME: 5 minutes
COOK TIME: —

1. In each of two small containers, layer one-quarter of the yogurt, flaxseed, cinnamon, berries, pumpkin seeds, and mint. Repeat the layers.

2. Serve, or store in the refrigerator for later in the week.

2 cups full-fat plain Greek yogurt

¼ cup ground flaxseed

1 teaspoon ground cinnamon

½ cup fresh blueberries

½ cup fresh raspberries

½ cup sliced fresh strawberries √

¼ cup shelled pumpkin seeds (pepitas)

¼ cup chopped fresh mint √

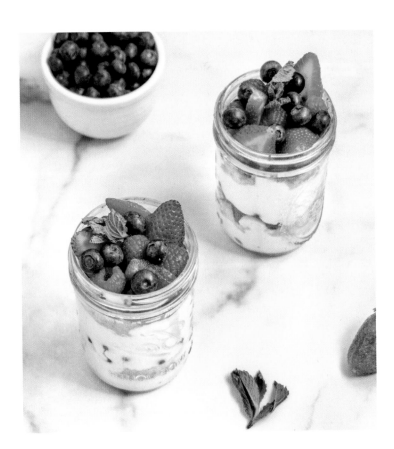

Overnight Protein Oats
with STRAWBERRY CHIA JAM

YIELD: 2 servings
PREP TIME: 5 minutes
COOK TIME: —

¾ cup old-fashioned oats

¼ cup (2 scoops) unflavored or vanilla-flavored protein powder

2 tablespoons ground flaxseed

½ teaspoon ground cinnamon

1 cup unsweetened nondairy milk of choice

1 cup fresh strawberries

1 tablespoon lemon juice

2 teaspoons maple syrup

1 tablespoon chia seeds

1. In a medium bowl, stir together the oats, protein powder, flaxseed, cinnamon, and milk. Cover and refrigerate at least overnight.

2. Make the jam: Dice the strawberries. In a small saucepan over low heat, cook the berries, lemon juice, maple syrup, and chia seeds, stirring frequently, for 5 minutes. Remove from the heat and let cool. The jam will continue to thicken as it cools.

3. Serve the oats topped with the jam.

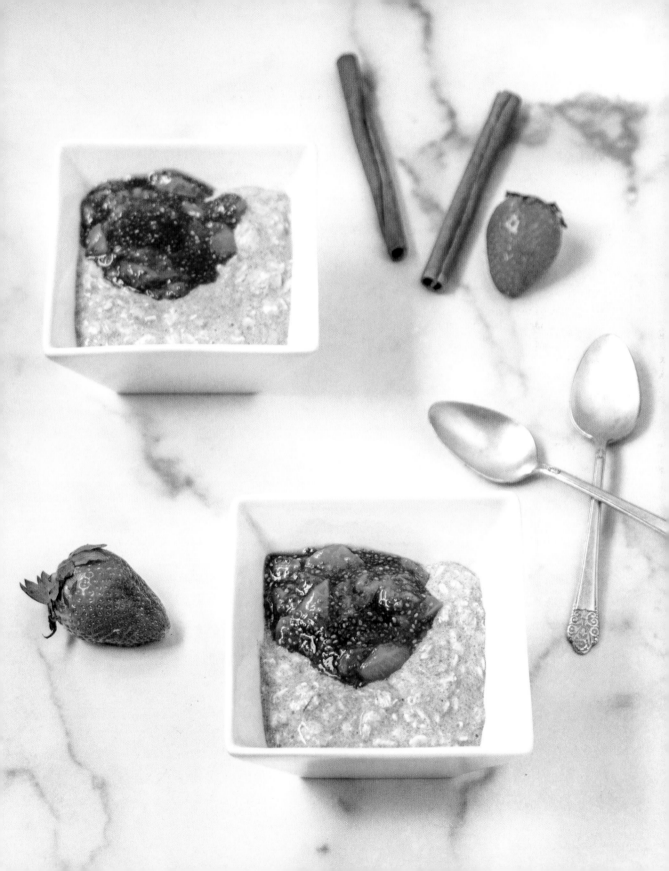

YIELD: 2 servings
PREP TIME: 5 minutes
COOK TIME: —

Deconstructed
SUMMER ROLL SALAD

2 cups mixed greens

2 (4-ounce) salmon fillets, baked √

1 cup cooked brown rice noodles √

1 cup shredded red cabbage √

1 cup sliced cucumbers √

4 radishes, sliced √

1 carrot, julienned √

4 green onions, thinly sliced √

½ Hass avocado, sliced

¼ cup shelled pumpkin seeds (pepitas)

¼ cup chopped fresh basil

¼ cup chopped fresh mint √

2 tablespoons avocado oil

1 tablespoon rice vinegar

1 tablespoon lime juice

Salt and pepper

1. Divide the greens evenly between two serving bowls.

2. Top the greens with the salmon, rice noodles, cabbage, cucumbers, radishes, carrot, green onions, avocado, pumpkin seeds, basil, and mint.

3. Make the dressing: In a small bowl, whisk together the oil, vinegar, lime juice, and salt and pepper to taste. Drizzle the dressing over the salads and serve.

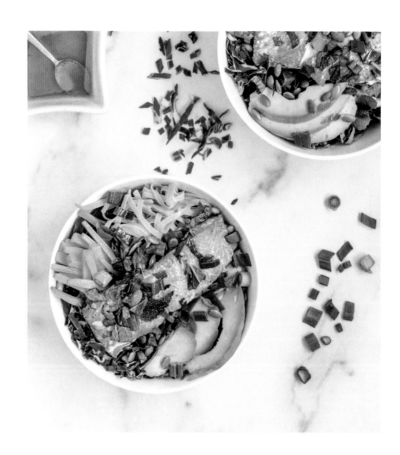

Summer
SALMON SALAD

YIELD: 2 servings
PREP TIME: 5 minutes
COOK TIME: —

1. In a large bowl, combine the greens with the oil and season with salt and pepper to taste. Divide the greens evenly between two serving bowls.

2. Top the greens with the salmon, strawberries, radishes, green onions, mint, pumpkin seeds, and goat cheese, if using.

3. Drizzle the balsamic glaze over the salads and serve.

2 cups mixed greens

2 tablespoons extra-virgin olive oil

Salt and pepper

2 (4-ounce) salmon fillets, baked √

1½ cups sliced fresh strawberries √

4 radishes, sliced √

2 green onions, thinly sliced √

¼ cup chopped fresh mint √

¼ cup shelled pumpkin seeds (pepitas)

2 ounces goat cheese, crumbled (optional)

2 teaspoons balsamic glaze

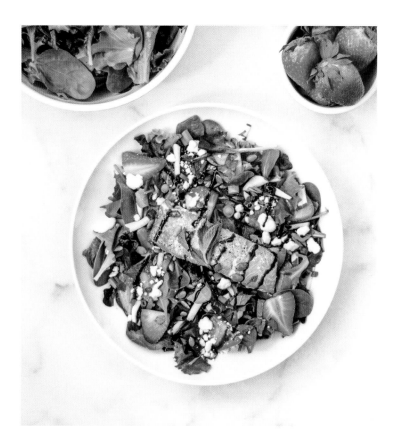

YIELD: 2 servings
PREP TIME: 10 minutes
COOK TIME: 8 minutes

Salmon with
PINEAPPLE-MINT SALSA

2 tablespoons avocado oil, divided

2 (4-ounce) salmon fillets

Salt and pepper

4 cups mixed greens

4 cups Pineapple-Mint Salsa √

1 Hass avocado, diced

1 cup canned black beans, drained and rinsed

¼ cup shelled pumpkin seeds (pepitas)

1. Heat 1 tablespoon of the oil in a large skillet over medium-high heat. Add the salmon and cook for 3 to 4 minutes on each side, until opaque in the center. Season with salt and pepper to taste.

2. Divide the greens evenly between two serving bowls. Top with the salsa, salmon, avocado, black beans, and pumpkin seeds and serve.

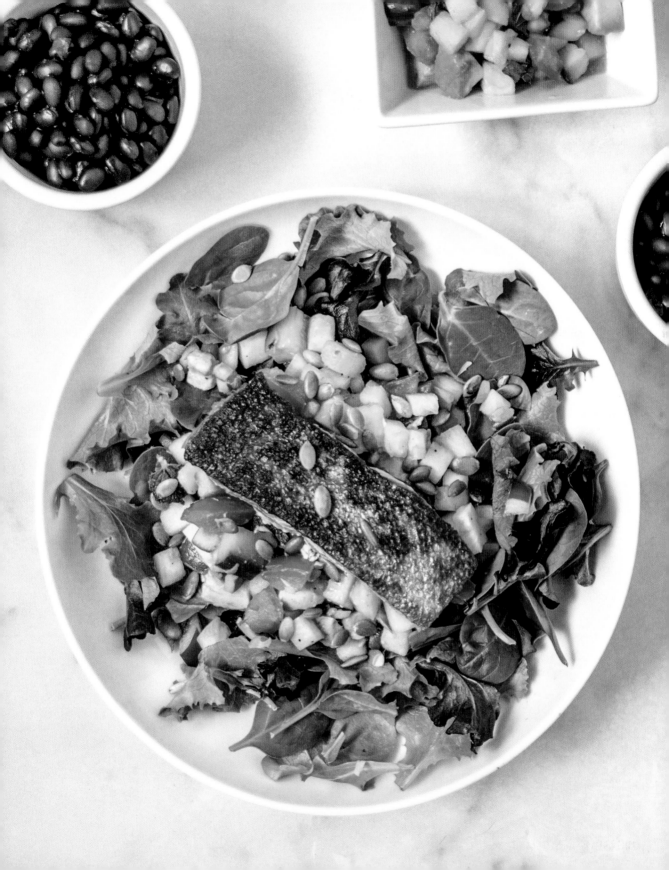

Pumpkin-Crusted
SALMON SHEET PAN DINNER

YIELD: 2 servings
PREP TIME: 10 minutes
COOK TIME: 25 minutes

½ cup shelled pumpkin seeds (pepitas)

2 cloves garlic, minced √

⅛ teaspoon fine sea salt

2 (4-ounce) salmon fillets

2 cups broccolini

1 cup baby red potatoes, halved

1 cup cherry tomatoes

1 tablespoon avocado oil

Ground black pepper

1. Preheat the oven to 375°F. Line a sheet pan with parchment paper or spray it with cooking spray.

2. Put the pumpkin seeds, garlic, and salt in a blender and blend to pulverize the seeds.

3. Place the salmon fillets on the prepared pan and pat the pumpkin seed mixture onto the top of each fillet.

4. Arrange the broccolini, potatoes, and tomatoes around the salmon. Drizzle with the oil and season with salt and pepper.

5. Bake for 25 minutes, until the salmon is opaque in the center and the vegetables are golden brown. Remove from the oven and serve, or store in the refrigerator for later in the week.

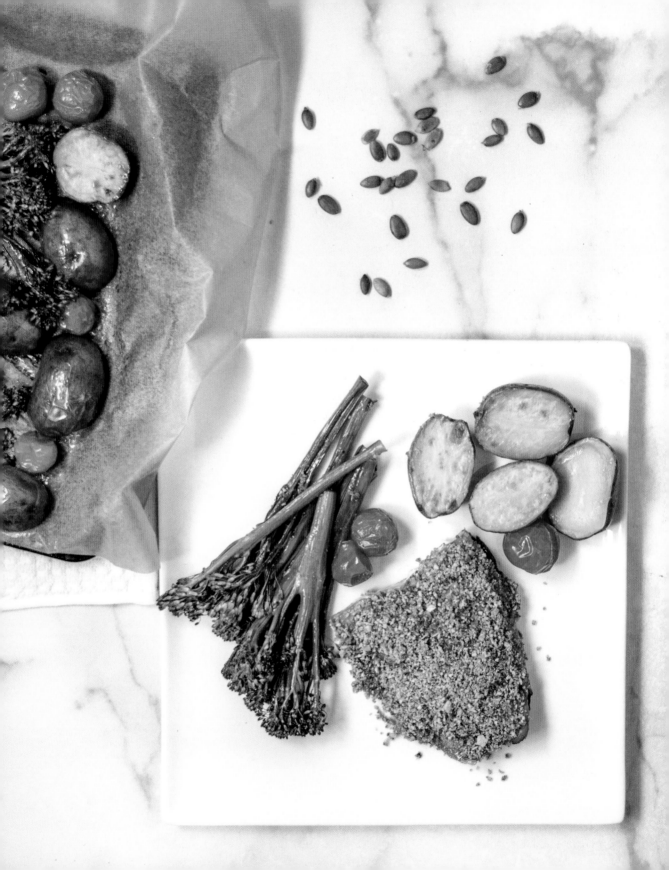

Week 11:

CHICKEN BREAST, CASHEWS, BLUEBERRIES, AND CILANTRO

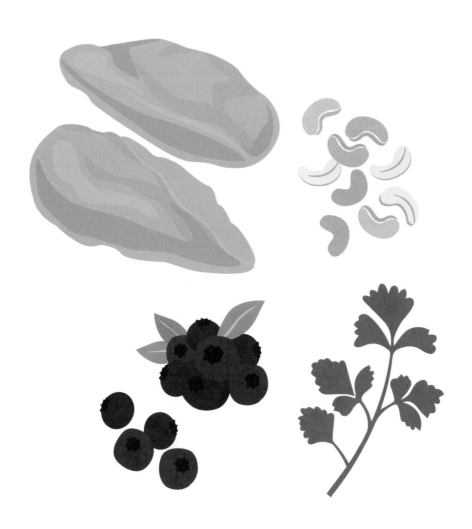

MENU

BREAKFAST	1	Blueberry Protein Muffins
	2	CB&J Overnight Oats
LUNCH	1	Thai Chicken Salad with Cashew Dressing
	2	Summer Chicken Salad
DINNER	1	Chimichurri Chicken with Coconut Cauliflower Rice
	2	Chicken Tacos with Blueberries

FEATURED INGREDIENTS

 ## PROTEIN

This week's protein is chicken breast, which is a lean source of protein. A 3.5-ounce serving has 115 calories and provides 21 grams of protein with less than 3 grams of fat. Chicken breast contains several nutrients beneficial for PCOS, including vitamins B6 and B12, iron, and magnesium.

 ## FIBER

Blueberries are this week's main source of fiber. One cup of blueberries provides nearly 4 grams of fiber and has only 85 calories. Blueberries are also high in anti-inflammatory antioxidants called anthocyanins and are a good source of many nutrients, including vitamin C.

 ## FAT

This week's fat is cashews, which are a good source of healthy monounsaturated fats and protein and are high in nutrients important for PCOS, such as magnesium, zinc, and folate.

 ## PCOS POWER FOOD

This week's PCOS Power Food is cilantro. Animal studies have suggested that cilantro may help lower blood sugar levels, and cilantro is high in inflammation-fighting antioxidants. Fresh cilantro is an easy and flavorful way to add nutrients to your meals.

WEEKLY INGREDIENTS

FRESH PRODUCE

Avocados, Hass, 2

Blueberries, 2 pints

Cauliflower, 1 head

Cilantro, 1 bunch

Coleslaw mix, 3 cups

Cucumbers, 2

Garlic, 6 cloves

Green onions, 6

Jalapeño pepper, 1

Radishes, 4

Red onion, 1

Romaine lettuce, 2 heads

MEAT/SEAFOOD

Chicken breasts, boneless, skinless,
2 pounds

EGGS/DAIRY/MILK

Eggs, 4 large

Unsweetened nondairy milk of choice,
1½ cups

PANTRY

Avocado oil, 2 tablespoons

Baking powder, 1 teaspoon

Cashew butter, ½ cup

Cashews, ½ cup

Chia seeds, 1 tablespoon

Coconut flakes, unsweetened,
2 tablespoons

Coconut flour, ½ cup

Coconut oil, ¼ cup

Corn tortillas, soft, 6-inch, 6

Ground flaxseed, ¼ cup

Lemon juice, 1 tablespoon

Lime juice, ½ cup

Maple syrup, 3 tablespoons

Old-fashioned oats, ¾ cup

Olive oil, extra-virgin, ¼ cup plus
2 tablespoons

Protein powder, unflavored or vanilla-
flavored, ½ cup (4 scoops)

Tamari, 1 tablespoon

Vanilla extract, 1 teaspoon

SEASONINGS

Ginger powder, ½ teaspoon

Ground cinnamon, ½ teaspoon

SUMMER

CUSTOMIZING THE PLAN

TO ADD MORE CARBS:

- Double the oats.
- Use whole-wheat flour in place of coconut flour in the Blueberry Protein Muffins.
- Replace the riced cauliflower with cooked brown rice in the Chimichurri Chicken.
- Add cooked brown rice, quinoa, or noodles to the lunch salads.

PREP DAY

Today you will be making the cashew dressing and chimichurri, cooking some of the chicken, and prepping some of the vegetables for the week. Also bake the Blueberry Protein Muffins and prepare the CB&J Overnight Oats.

Complete the following tasks and store each component in a separate container in the refrigerator for use later in the week.

MAKE THE CASHEW DRESSING

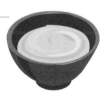

YIELD: ½ cup
PREP TIME: 5 minutes
COOK TIME: —

Put ¼ cup cashew butter, 2 tablespoons water, 1 tablespoon lime juice, 1 tablespoon tamari, 1 clove garlic (peeled), and ½ teaspoon ginger powder in a blender and blend until smooth.

MAKE THE CHIMICHURRI SAUCE

YIELD: 1 cup
PREP TIME: 5 minutes
COOK TIME: —

Put 1 cup fresh cilantro, ¼ cup lime juice, ¼ cup extra-virgin olive oil, 2 cloves garlic (peeled), and ⅛ teaspoon fine sea salt in a blender and blend until combined.

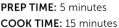

COOK SOME OF THE CHICKEN

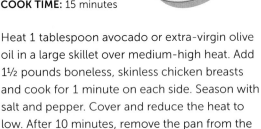

PREP TIME: 5 minutes
COOK TIME: 15 minutes

Heat 1 tablespoon avocado or extra-virgin olive oil in a large skillet over medium-high heat. Add 1½ pounds boneless, skinless chicken breasts and cook for 1 minute on each side. Season with salt and pepper. Cover and reduce the heat to low. After 10 minutes, remove the pan from the heat and let sit covered for another 10 minutes. Slice the chicken into strips.

SLICE THE RADISHES

Thinly slice 4 radishes.

CHOP THE CILANTRO

Chop enough fresh cilantro to measure 1 cup.

SLICE THE GREEN ONIONS

Thinly slice 6 green onions.

CHOP THE LETTUCE

Chop enough romaine lettuce to measure 4 cups.

RICE THE CAULIFLOWER

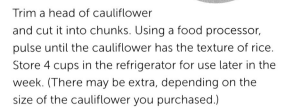

Trim a head of cauliflower and cut it into chunks. Using a food processor, pulse until the cauliflower has the texture of rice. Store 4 cups in the refrigerator for use later in the week. (There may be extra, depending on the size of the cauliflower you purchased.)

DICE THE RED ONION

Dice enough red onion to measure ¼ cup.

SLICE THE JALAPEÑO

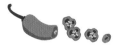

Slice 1 jalapeño pepper and remove the seeds, if desired.

MINCE THE REST OF THE GARLIC

Mince 3 cloves of garlic.

SLICE THE CUCUMBER

Slice enough cucumber to measure 2 cups.

Blueberry
PROTEIN MUFFINS

YIELD: 8 muffins (2 per serving)
PREP TIME: 5 minutes
COOK TIME: 25 minutes

1. Preheat the oven to 350°F and spray 8 wells of a standard-size muffin tin with cooking spray.

2. In a large bowl, whisk together the coconut flour, protein powder, flaxseed, baking powder, and salt.

3. Add the eggs, milk, coconut oil, maple syrup, and vanilla and stir to combine.

4. Gently fold the blueberries into the batter.

5. Scoop the batter into the prepared wells of the muffin tin, filling them two-thirds full. Bake for 22 to 25 minutes, until a toothpick inserted in the center of a muffin comes out clean.

6. Remove from the oven, transfer the muffins to a cooling rack, and let cool. Serve, or store in the fridge for later in the week.

½ cup coconut flour

¼ cup (2 scoops) unflavored or vanilla-flavored protein powder

2 tablespoons ground flaxseed

1 teaspoon baking powder

⅛ teaspoon fine sea salt

4 large eggs

½ cup unsweetened nondairy milk of choice

¼ cup coconut oil, melted

2 tablespoons maple syrup

1 teaspoon vanilla extract

1 cup fresh blueberries

NOTE:
These muffins freeze well, so you can freeze any leftovers that you do not plan on eating within the week.

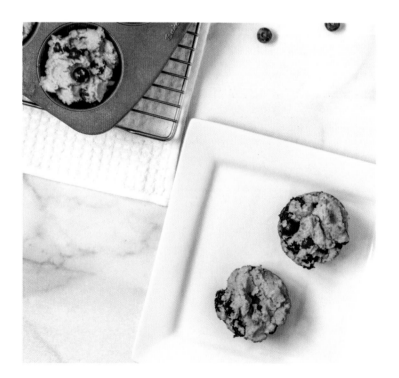

YIELD: 2 servings
PREP TIME: 5 minutes
COOK TIME: —

CB&J
OVERNIGHT OATS

¾ cup old-fashioned oats

¼ cup (2 scoops) unflavored or vanilla-flavored protein powder

2 tablespoons ground flaxseed

½ teaspoon ground cinnamon

1 cup unsweetened nondairy milk of choice

1 cup fresh blueberries

1 tablespoon chia seeds

1 tablespoon lemon juice

2 teaspoons maple syrup

2 tablespoons cashew butter

1. In a medium bowl, stir together the oats, protein powder, flaxseed, cinnamon, and milk. Cover and refrigerate at least overnight.

2. Make the jam: In a small saucepan over low heat, combine the blueberries, chia seeds, lemon juice, and maple syrup and cook, stirring frequently, for 5 minutes. Remove from the heat and let cool. The jam will continue to thicken as it cools.

3. Serve the oats topped with the jam and cashew butter.

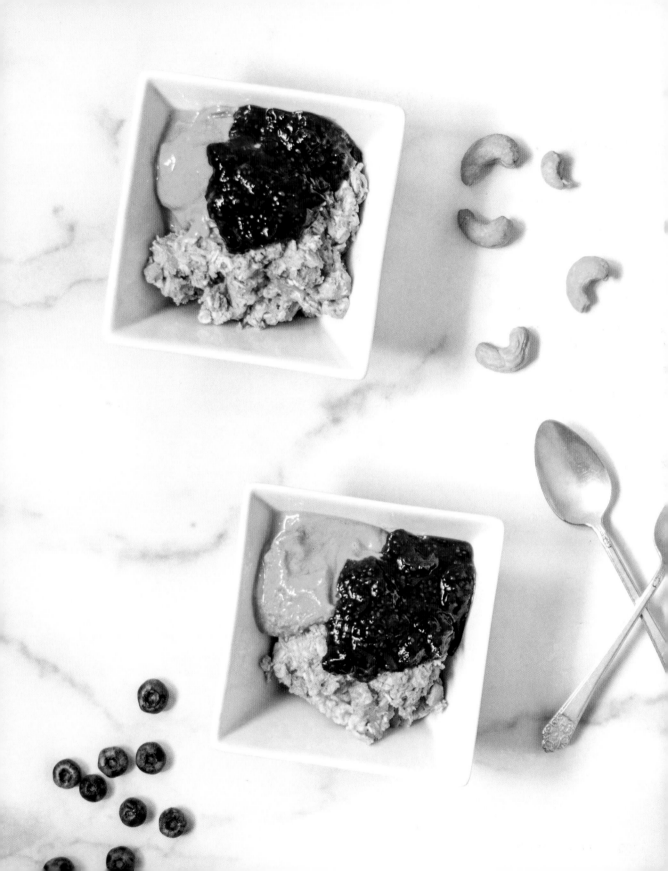

Thai Chicken Salad with
CASHEW DRESSING

YIELD: 2 servings
PREP TIME: 5 minutes
COOK TIME: —

2 cups coleslaw mix

One-third of the cooked and sliced chicken breast √

1 cup sliced cucumbers √

4 radishes, sliced √

½ Hass avocado, diced

2 green onions, thinly sliced √

½ cup chopped fresh cilantro √

½ cup Cashew Dressing √

1. Divide the coleslaw mix evenly between two serving bowls.

2. Top with the chicken, cucumbers, radishes, avocado, green onions, and cilantro.

3. Drizzle the dressing over the salads and serve.

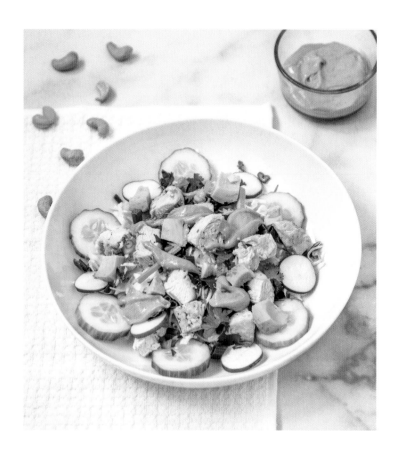

Summer
CHICKEN SALAD

YIELD: 2 servings
PREP TIME: 5 minutes
COOK TIME: —

1. Divide the lettuce evenly between two serving bowls.

2. Top with the chicken, blueberries, cucumbers, radishes, avocado, red onions, cashews, and cilantro.

3. Make the dressing: In a small bowl, whisk together the oil and lime juice and season with salt and pepper to taste. Drizzle the dressing over the salads and serve.

4 cups chopped romaine lettuce √

One-third of the cooked and sliced chicken breast √

1 cup fresh blueberries

1 cup sliced cucumbers √

4 radishes, sliced √

½ Hass avocado, diced

¼ cup diced red onions √

¼ cup cashews

½ cup chopped fresh cilantro √

2 tablespoons extra-virgin olive oil

2 tablespoons lime juice

Salt and pepper

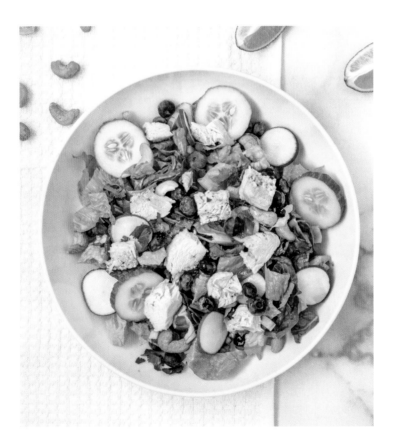

Chimichurri Chicken
with COCONUT CAULIFLOWER RICE

YIELD: 2 servings
PREP TIME: 5 minutes
COOK TIME: 20 minutes

2 tablespoons avocado oil, divided

2 (4-ounce) boneless, skinless chicken breasts

4 cups riced cauliflower √

¼ cup cashews

2 tablespoons unsweetened flaked coconut

2 green onions, thinly sliced √

½ cup Chimichurri Sauce √

Salt and pepper

1. Heat 1 tablespoon of the oil in a large skillet over medium-high heat. Add the chicken and cook for 4 to 5 minutes on each side, until no longer pink in the center.

2. Meanwhile, heat the remaining tablespoon of oil in another large skillet over medium-high heat. Add the riced cauliflower and cook, stirring frequently, until softened, about 5 minutes.

3. Add the cashews, coconut, and green onions to the pan with the cauliflower and stir to combine.

4. Divide the cauliflower rice evenly between two serving plates, top with the chicken, and drizzle the chimichurri sauce over the chicken.

5. Serve, or store in the refrigerator for later in the week.

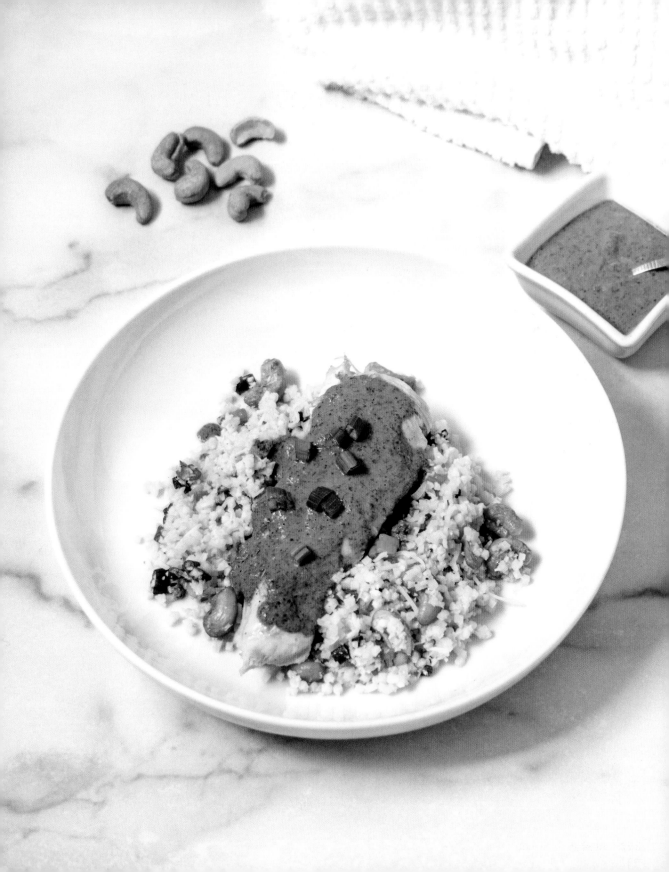

YIELD: 2 servings
PREP TIME: 10 minutes
COOK TIME: 5 minutes

Chicken Tacos
with BLUEBERRIES

6 (6-inch) soft corn tortillas

1 cup coleslaw mix

One-third of the cooked and sliced chicken breast √

½ Hass avocado, diced

½ cup fresh blueberries

1 jalapeño pepper, sliced √

2 green onions, thinly sliced √

½ cup Chimichurri Sauce √

1. Warm the tortillas in a small dry skillet over low heat. Place 3 tortillas on each of two serving plates.

2. Layer the coleslaw mix, chicken, avocado, blueberries, jalapeño slices, and green onions on the tortillas.

3. Drizzle the tacos with the chimichurri sauce and serve.

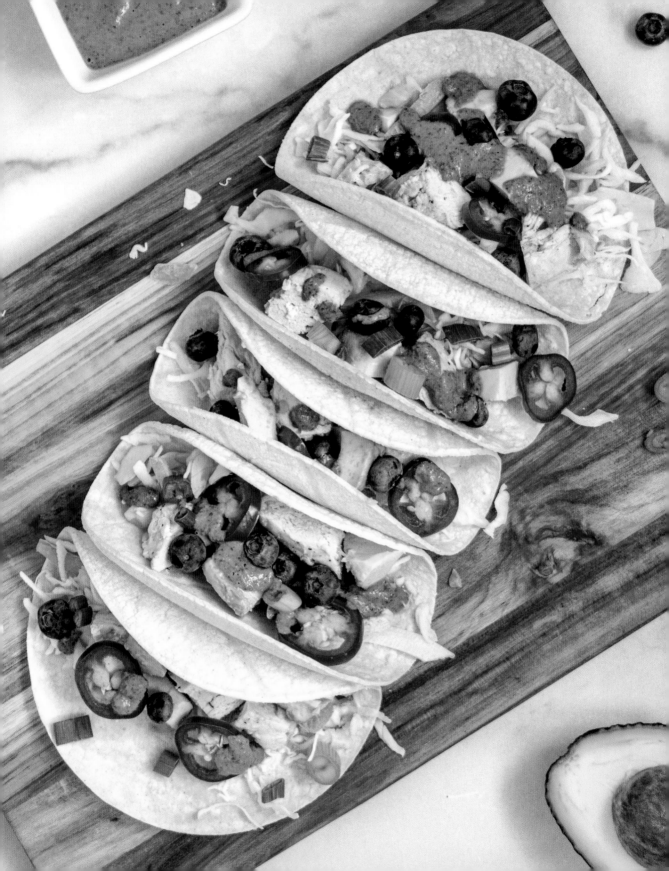

Week 12:

GROUND BEEF, OLIVE OIL, MUSHROOMS, AND CAULIFLOWER

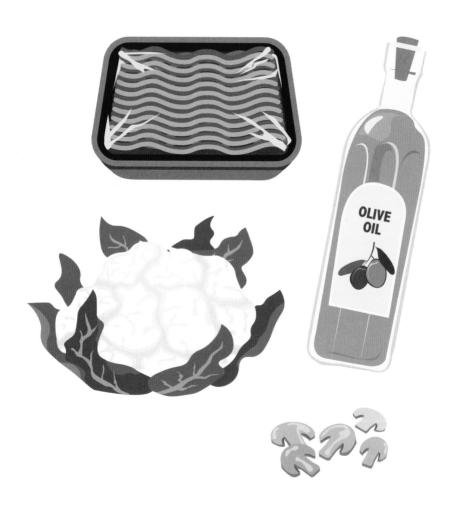

MENU

BREAKFAST	1	Egg Pepper Cups
	2	Mushroom Mini Quiches
LUNCH	1	Summer Veggie Chili with Beef
	2	Beef Burrito Bowls
DINNER	1	Burger Salad
	2	Unstuffed Peppers

FEATURED INGREDIENTS

PROTEIN

This week's protein is ground beef, which is a good source of protein and nutrients. One serving provides nearly one-third of your daily vitamin B12 needs and 10 percent of your daily iron needs. If you want to eat less fat, you can look for 90 percent lean ground beef; otherwise, use 85 or 80 percent lean.

FIBER

Mushrooms contribute fiber to this week's menu. One cup of mushrooms has about 1 gram of fiber and has only 16 calories. Mushrooms also have vitamin D and some B vitamins and vitamin C. They add a meaty flavor and help cut down on the amount of meat used in recipes.

FAT

This week's fat is olive oil, which is a staple of the anti-inflammatory Mediterranean diet. Extra-virgin olive oil is not only safe to cook with but adds a delicious flavor to almost any dish.

PCOS POWER FOOD

This week's PCOS Power Food is cauliflower. Cauliflower is low in calories and carbs and high in fiber and nutrients, including vitamin C, vitamin B6, and magnesium. Cruciferous vegetables such as cauliflower help the liver do its job in detoxing hormones such as estrogen, making them a smart choice for PCOS. Cauliflower is also a good source of antioxidants, which can help with inflammation.

WEEKLY INGREDIENTS

FRESH PRODUCE

Avocado, Hass, 1

Button mushrooms, whole or sliced, 12 ounces

Cauliflower, 1 large head

Cherry tomatoes, 2½ cups

Garlic, 5 cloves

Green bell peppers, 3

Green leaf lettuce, 4 cups

Green onions, 2

Orange or yellow bell pepper, 1

Red bell peppers, 2

Red onion, 1

Shallots, ½ cup

Yellow onions, 2

Zucchini, 1

MEAT/SEAFOOD

Ground beef, 2 pounds

EGGS/DAIRY/MILK

Cheddar cheese, 2 ounces (optional, for Egg Pepper Cups)

Eggs, 12 large

Greek yogurt, full-fat plain, ½ cup

Unsweetened nondairy milk of choice, 2 tablespoons

PANTRY

Black beans, 1 (15-ounce) can

Diced tomatoes, 2 (15-ounce) cans

Dijon mustard, 2 teaspoons

Dill pickle spears, 2

Lime juice, 2 tablespoons

Olive oil, extra-virgin, ½ cup plus 2 tablespoons

Pinto beans, 1 (15-ounce) can

Sriracha sauce, 1 teaspoon

SEASONINGS

Chili powder, 3 tablespoons

Dried parsley, 1 teaspoon

CUSTOMIZING THE PLAN

TO ADD MORE CARBS:

- Substitute cooked brown rice for the riced cauliflower in the Summer Veggie Chili, Unstuffed Peppers, and Burrito Bowls.

- Have a piece of whole-wheat bread or add cooked brown rice or quinoa to the Burger Salad.

- Have a piece of toast with the Egg Pepper Cups and Mushroom Mini Quiches.

TO MAKE THIS WEEK DAIRY-FREE:

- Omit the cheese from the Egg Pepper Cups.

- Use a nondairy yogurt in place of the Greek yogurt.

PREP DAY

Today you will be cooking some of the ground beef and riced cauliflower and prepping some of the vegetables for the week. Make the Egg Pepper Cups and the Mushroom Mini Quiches as well.

Complete the following tasks and store each component in a separate container in the refrigerator for use later in the week.

COOK SOME OF THE GROUND BEEF

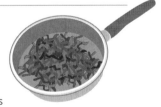

PREP TIME: 5 minutes
COOK TIME: 10 minutes

In a large skillet over medium-high heat, cook 1 pound ground beef, breaking up the meat into smaller pieces, until no longer pink, about 10 minutes. Season with salt and pepper to taste. Store half for use in the Burger Salad. To the other half of the beef, add 1 tablespoon chili powder and store for use in the Burrito Bowls.

RICE THE CAULIFLOWER

Trim a large head of cauliflower and cut it into chunks. Using a food processor, pulse until the cauliflower has the texture of rice. Set 2 cups aside to cook today, and store 4 cups in the refrigerator for use later in the week. (There may be extra, depending on the size of the head of cauliflower you purchased.)

COOK THE RICED CAULIFLOWER

Put 2 cups riced cauliflower in a medium skillet with 1 tablespoon extra-virgin olive oil and season with salt and pepper. Cook until soft, about 5 minutes.

DICE THE YELLOW AND RED ONIONS

Dice enough yellow onions to measure 2 cups and enough red onion to measure ½ cup. Store separately.

DICE THE SHALLOTS

Finely dice enough shallots to measure ½ cup.

DICE THE BELL PEPPERS

Dice 1 green bell pepper, 1 orange or yellow bell pepper, and 1 red bell pepper and store together in the refrigerator for use in the Unstuffed Peppers. Dice an additional green bell pepper and store separately for use in the chili.

HALVE THE TOMATOES

Halve enough cherry tomatoes to measure ½ cup.

DICE THE ZUCCHINI

Dice enough zucchini to measure 1 cup.

SLICE THE MUSHROOMS

Slice enough mushrooms to measure 3 cups. (If you bought presliced mushrooms, skip this step.)

CHOP THE CILANTRO

Chop enough fresh cilantro to measure ½ cup.

MINCE THE GARLIC

Mince 8 cloves of garlic.

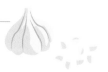

SLICE THE GREEN ONIONS

Thinly slice 2 green onions.

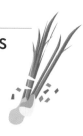

Egg Pepper
CUPS

YIELD: 2 servings
PREP TIME: 5 minutes
COOK TIME: 35 minutes

1. Preheat the oven to 400°F.

2. Slice the bell peppers in half lengthwise and remove the seeds and ribs. Place the pepper halves cut side up on a sheet pan.

3. Crack an egg into each pepper cup. Season with salt and pepper.

4. Bake for 30 minutes, or until the eggs are set. Remove from the oven.

5. If using cheese, sprinkle the cheese over the eggs and place the pan under the broiler for 3 to 5 minutes, until the cheese is melted.

6. Serve, or store in the refrigerator for later in the week.

1 green bell pepper

1 red bell pepper

4 large eggs

Salt and pepper

2 ounces cheddar cheese, shredded (optional)

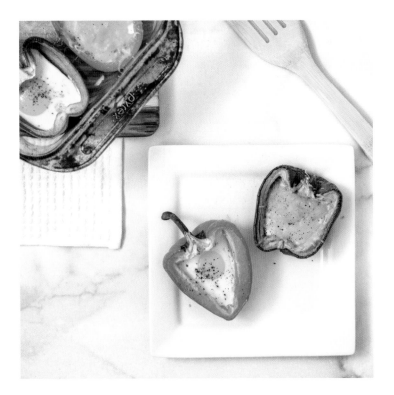

YIELD: 4 mini quiches (2 per serving)
PREP TIME: 5 minutes
COOK TIME: 28 minutes

Mushroom
MINI QUICHES

½ cup finely diced shallots √

1 tablespoon extra-virgin olive oil

2 cups sliced button mushrooms √

1 clove garlic, minced √

1 teaspoon dried parsley

4 large eggs

4 large egg whites

2 tablespoons unsweetened nondairy milk of choice

Salt and pepper

1. Preheat the oven to 350°F and spray four 4-ounce ramekins with cooking spray.

2. In a medium skillet over medium-high heat, sauté the shallots in the oil until soft, about 3 minutes. Add the mushrooms and sauté until softened and starting to brown, about 5 minutes. Stir in the garlic and parsley.

3. Meanwhile, in a medium bowl, whisk together the whole eggs, egg whites, and milk. Season with salt and pepper.

4. Pour the egg mixture evenly into the ramekins, then divide the mushroom mixture evenly among the ramekins.

5. Bake for 20 minutes, or until the eggs are set. Serve, or store in the refrigerator for later in the week.

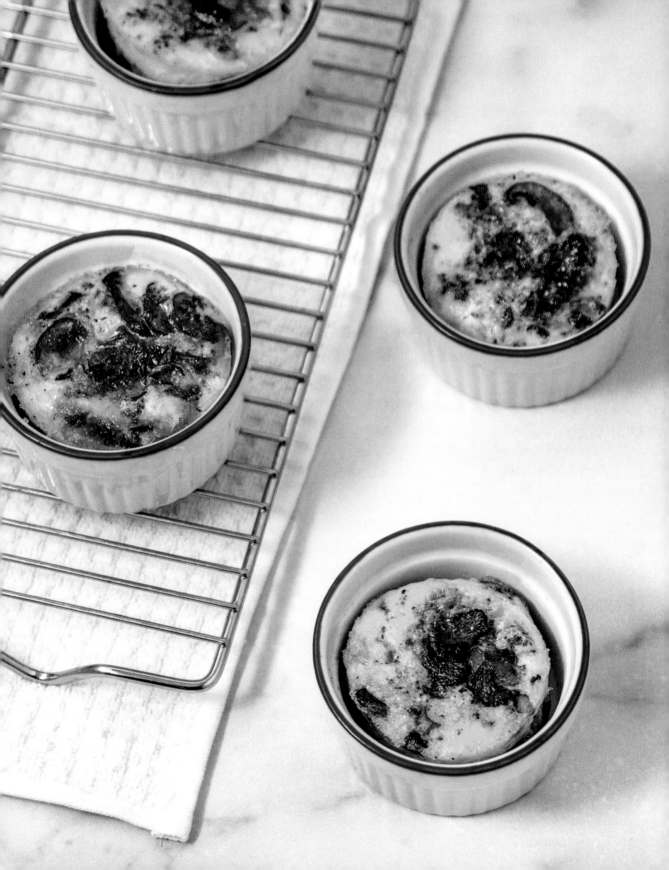

YIELD: 2 servings
PREP TIME: 5 minutes
COOK TIME: 25 minutes

Summer Veggie Chili
with BEEF

1 cup diced yellow onions √

2 tablespoons extra-virgin olive oil

8 ounces ground beef

2 cups riced cauliflower √

1 cup diced green bell peppers √

1 cup sliced button mushrooms √

1 cup diced zucchini √

1 (15-ounce) can diced tomatoes

1 (15-ounce) can pinto beans, drained and rinsed

2 cloves garlic, minced √

2 tablespoons chili powder

Salt and pepper

NOTE:
This chili freezes well, so you can freeze any leftovers that you do not plan on eating within the week.

1. In a large pot over medium-high heat, sauté the onions in the oil until soft, about 5 minutes.

2. Add the ground beef and cook, breaking it up with a spatula, until no longer pink, about 5 minutes.

3. Add the riced cauliflower, bell peppers, mushrooms, zucchini, tomatoes, pinto beans, garlic, and chili powder to the pot. Cover, reduce the heat to medium-low, and simmer until all the vegetables are tender, 10 to 15 minutes.

4. Season the chili with salt and pepper and serve, or store in the refrigerator for later in the week.

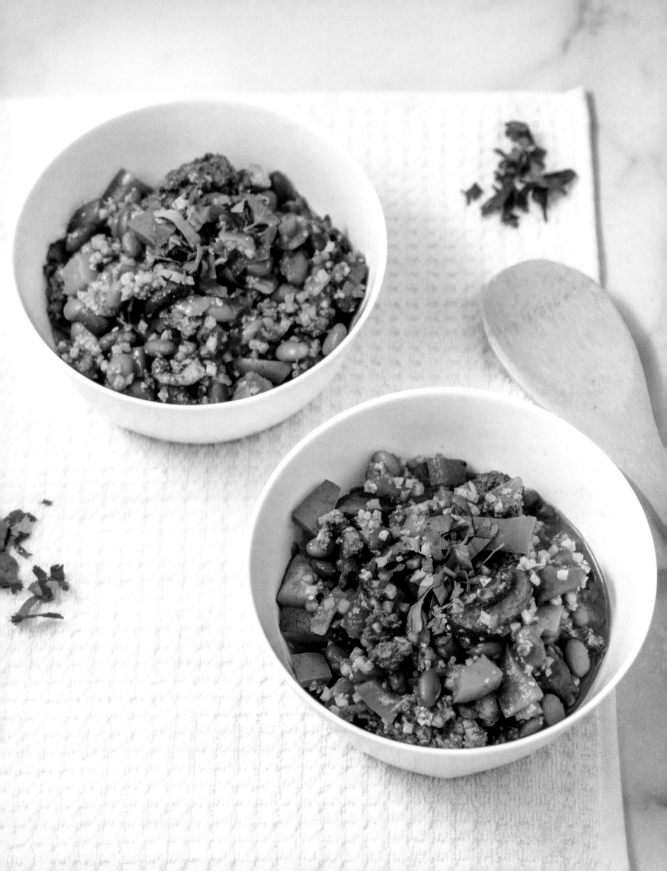

Beef Burrito
BOWLS

YIELD: 2 servings
PREP TIME: 5 minutes
COOK TIME: —

2 cups riced cauliflower, cooked √

Half of the cooked and seasoned ground beef √

1 (15-ounce) can black beans, drained and rinsed

½ cup cherry tomatoes, halved √

½ Hass avocado, diced

2 green onions, thinly sliced √

½ cup chopped fresh cilantro √

2 tablespoons extra-virgin olive oil

2 tablespoons lime juice

Salt and pepper

1. Divide the riced cauliflower evenly between two serving bowls.

2. Top with the ground beef, black beans, tomatoes, avocado, green onions, and cilantro.

3. Make the dressing: In a small bowl, combine the oil and lime juice and season with salt and pepper to taste. Drizzle the dressing over the bowls and serve.

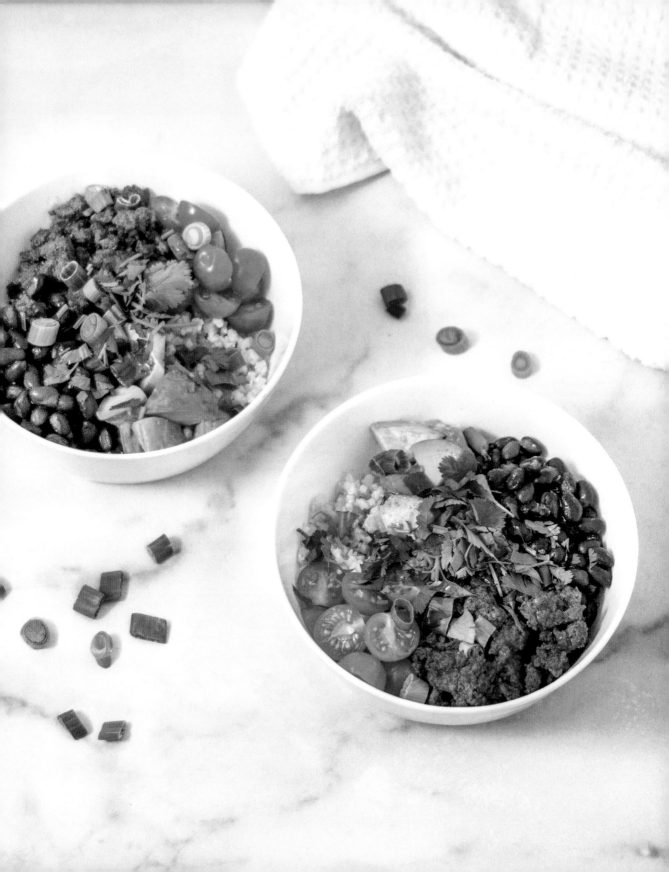

YIELD: 2 servings
PREP TIME: 5 minutes
COOK TIME: 15 minutes

Burger
SALAD

4 cups chopped green leaf lettuce

Half of the cooked and seasoned ground beef √

1 pint cherry tomatoes

½ cup diced red onions √

2 dill pickle spears, diced

½ cup plain full-fat Greek yogurt

2 tablespoons extra-virgin olive oil

2 teaspoons Dijon mustard

1 teaspoon Sriracha sauce

Salt and pepper

1. Divide the lettuce evenly between two serving plates. Top with the ground beef, tomatoes, onions, and pickles.

2. Make the dressing: In a small bowl, whisk together the yogurt, oil, mustard, and Sriracha. Drizzle the dressing over the salads, season with salt and pepper to taste, and serve.

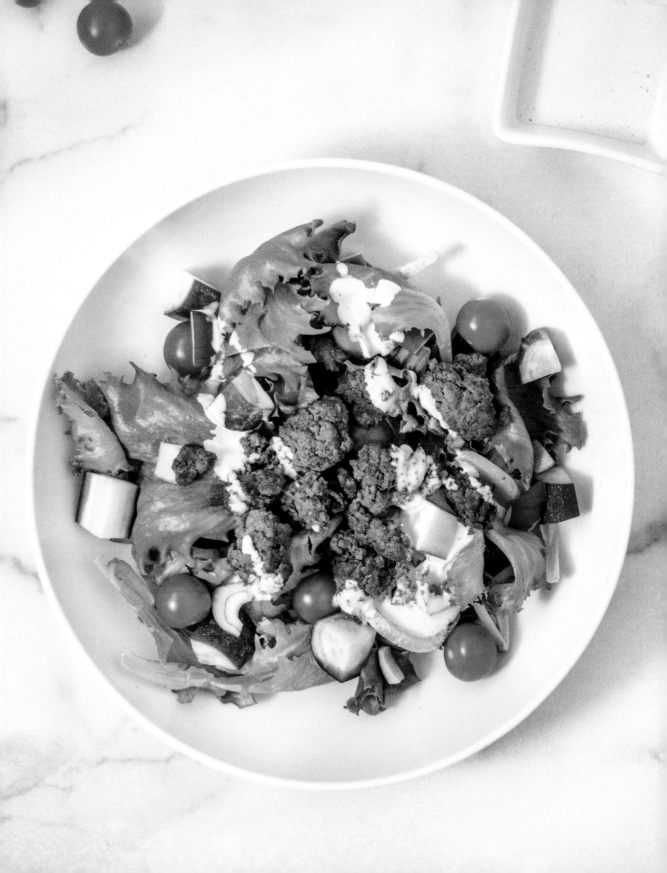

YIELD: 2 servings
PREP TIME: 5 minutes
COOK TIME: 25 minutes

Unstuffed
PEPPERS

1 cup diced yellow onions √

1 green bell pepper, diced √

1 yellow or orange bell pepper, diced √

1 red bell pepper, diced √

2 tablespoons extra-virgin olive oil

8 ounces ground beef

2 cups riced cauliflower √

2 cloves garlic, minced √

1 (15-ounce) can diced tomatoes

Salt and pepper

1. In a large skillet over medium-high heat, sauté the onions and bell peppers in the oil until soft, about 5 minutes.

2. At the same time, in a medium skillet over medium-high heat, cook the ground beef until no longer pink, about 10 minutes.

3. Add the riced cauliflower, garlic, and tomatoes to the pan with the ground beef. Stir to combine and cook until heated through, about 10 minutes. Season with salt and pepper to taste.

4. Divide the onions and peppers evenly between two plates, top with the beef mixture, and serve, or store in the refrigerator for later in the week.

NOTE:
This dish freezes well, so you can freeze any leftovers that you do not plan on eating within the week.

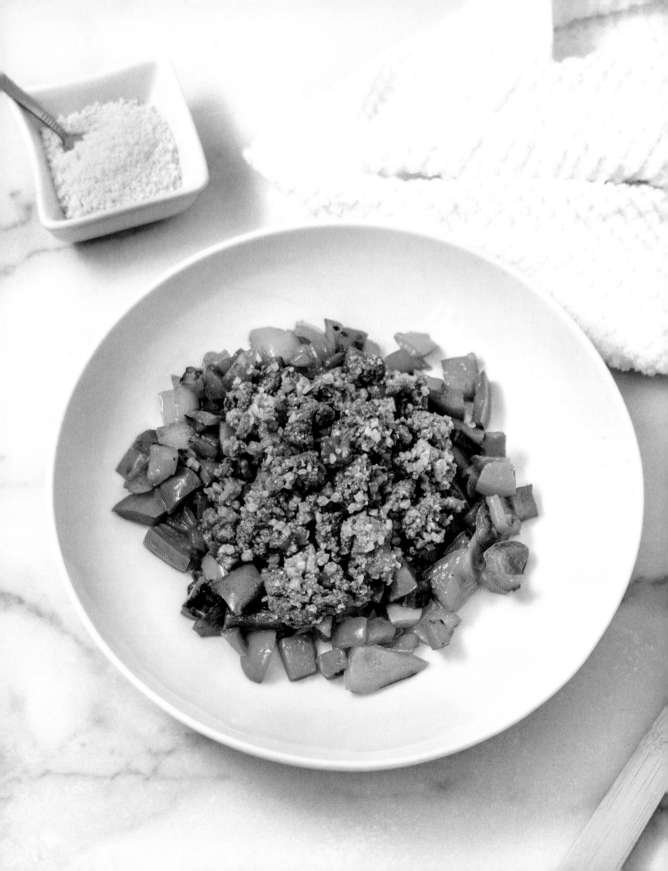

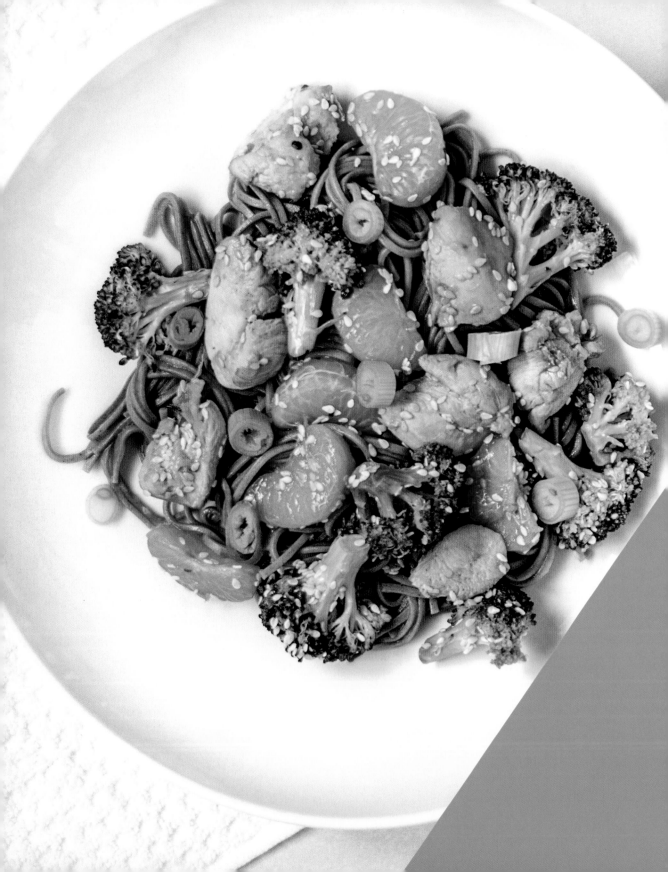

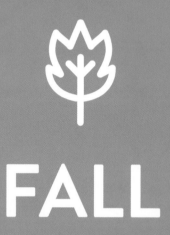

FALL

Week 13:

TUNA, PECANS, CHICKPEA PASTA, AND ARUGULA

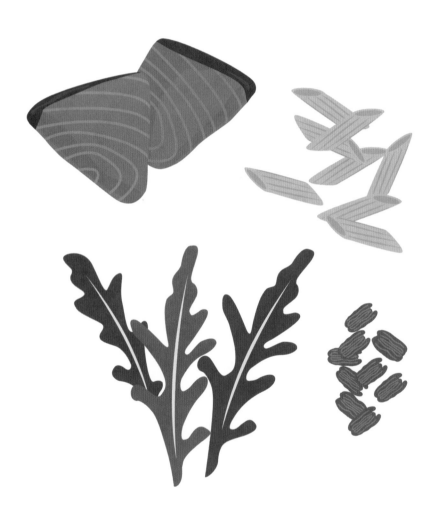

MENU

BREAKFAST	1	Breakfast Salad
	2	Pecan Pie Protein Muffins
LUNCH	1	Mediterranean Chickpea Pasta Salad
	2	Fall Tuna Salad
DINNER	1	Tuna Bolognese with Chickpea Pasta
	2	Seared Tuna with Arugula Pecan Pesto and Mashed Cauliflower

FEATURED INGREDIENTS

 ### PROTEIN

This week's protein is tuna, which is a lean source of protein that provides a small amount of anti-inflammatory omega-3 fatty acids. A 3-ounce serving of tuna canned in water has 100 calories and provides 22 grams of protein with less than 1 gram of fat. Tuna contains several nutrients beneficial for PCOS, including vitamins B6 and B12, niacin, choline, iron, and magnesium. While tuna is higher in mercury than many other types of fish, there are many canned tunas on the market that use low-mercury sourced fish. The current recommendation is that pregnant women should limit their consumption to 12 ounces of light tuna or 6 ounces of albacore tuna per week.

 ### FAT

This week's fat is pecans, which are a good source of healthy monounsaturated fats and protein and are high in nutrients important for PCOS, such as vitamin E, potassium, and zinc.

 ### FIBER

Chickpea pasta is this week's main source of fiber. Chickpea pasta is higher in protein and fiber and lower in carbs than whole-wheat pasta. One 2-ounce serving provides 5 grams of fiber. Most grocery stores carry several brands.

 ### PCOS POWER FOOD

This week's PCOS Power Food is arugula. Arugula is a cruciferous vegetable that may help your liver metabolize excess hormones. In addition, it is low in calories and high in antioxidants and nutrients, including folate, vitamins C and K, and beta-carotene.

WEEKLY INGREDIENTS

FRESH PRODUCE

Apple (any type), 1

Arugula, 11 cups

Avocado, Hass, 1

Carrot, 1

Cauliflower, 1 head

Celery, 3 stalks

Cucumber, 1

Garlic, 3 cloves

Kale, curly, 1 bunch

Parsley, curly or Italian, 1 bunch

Red grapefruit, 1

Red onion, 1

Yellow onion, 1

MEAT/SEAFOOD

Tuna steaks, 8 ounces

Turkey bacon, 4 slices

EGGS/DAIRY/MILK

Eggs, 8 large

Parmesan cheese, grated, ¼ cup plus 2 tablespoons (optional, for the pesto and the Bolognese)

Unsweetened nondairy milk of choice, ½ cup plus 2 tablespoons

SEASONINGS

Dried basil, 1 teaspoon

Ground cinnamon, ½ teaspoon

PANTRY

Artichoke hearts, quartered, packed in water, 1 (15-ounce) can

Baking powder, 1 teaspoon

Blackstrap molasses, 2 tablespoons

Capers, 2 tablespoons

Chickpea pasta, 2 (8-ounce) boxes

Coconut oil, ¼ cup

Cooking spray (avocado or olive oil)

Hemp seeds, hulled, 2 tablespoons

Kalamata olives, pitted, ¼ cup

Lemon juice, ½ cup

Olive oil, extra-virgin, ¾ cup

Pecan halves, raw, 2¼ cups

Raisins, ¼ cup

Sun-dried tomatoes, dried (not jarred), ¼ cup

Tomato paste, 2 tablespoons

Tomato sauce, 1 (15-ounce) can

Tuna packed in olive oil, 1 (5-ounce) can

Tuna packed in water, 2 (5-ounce) cans

Unflavored or vanilla-flavored protein powder, ¼ cup (2 scoops)

Vanilla extract, 1 teaspoon

White beans, 1 (15-ounce) can

Whole-grain mustard, ¼ cup

CUSTOMIZING THE PLAN

TO ADD MORE CARBS:

- Use whole-wheat pasta in place of the chickpea pasta and double the amounts used in the recipes.

- Use whole-wheat flour in place of the pecan flour in the Pecan Pie Protein Muffins.

- Replace the mashed cauliflower with mashed potatoes in the Seared Tuna recipe.

- Have a piece of whole-grain toast with the Breakfast Salad.

TO MAKE THIS WEEK DAIRY-FREE:

- Omit the Parmesan cheese.

PREP DAY

Today you will be making the mashed cauliflower and the pesto, cooking the pasta, eggs, and bacon, and prepping some of the vegetables for the week. Bake the Pecan Pie Protein Muffins (page 232) as well.

Complete the following tasks and store each component in a separate container in the refrigerator for use later in the week.

MINCE THE GARLIC

Mince 3 cloves of garlic. Set aside 1 clove for the mashed cauliflower and store the rest for use later in the week.

COOK THE PASTA

YIELD: 3 cups
PREP TIME: 5 minutes
COOK TIME: 10 minutes

Cook 3 cups chickpea pasta according to the package directions. Drain and rinse.

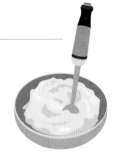

MAKE THE MASHED CAULIFLOWER

YIELD: about 2 cups
PREP TIME: 10 minutes
COOK TIME: 10 minutes

Trim and roughly chop a head of cauliflower and place it in a large pot. Add 1 inch of water and bring to a boil over medium-high heat. Once the cauliflower is tender, about 10 minutes, remove the pot from the heat and drain the water. Add 2 tablespoons unsweetened nondairy milk of choice, 1 clove minced garlic, and salt and pepper to taste. Mash the cauliflower using a potato masher or an immersion blender until smooth.

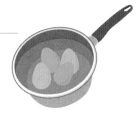

SOFT-BOIL SOME OF THE EGGS

PREP TIME: 2 minutes
COOK TIME: 6 minutes

Bring a small saucepan of water to a boil over medium-high heat. Carefully lower 4 eggs into the water and reduce the heat to a simmer. After 6 minutes, immediately remove the eggs from the hot water and place in a bowl of cold water for 10 minutes. When the eggs are cool, peel them.

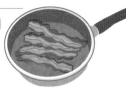

COOK THE BACON

PREP TIME: 5 minutes
COOK TIME: 8 minutes

In a large skillet over medium-high heat, cook 4 slices turkey bacon for 3 to 4 minutes per side, to the desired crispness.

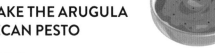

MAKE THE ARUGULA PECAN PESTO

YIELD: 2 cups
PREP TIME: 5 minutes
COOK TIME: —

1 cup arugula
1 cup fresh parsley
½ cup raw pecan halves
¼ cup extra-virgin olive oil
¼ cup grated Parmesan cheese (optional)

2 tablespoons lemon juice
1 clove garlic
¼ teaspoon fine sea salt

Put all of the ingredients in a food processor and pulse until smooth.

SLICE THE RED ONION

Thinly slice enough red onion to measure ¼ cup.

DICE THE CUCUMBER

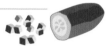

Dice enough cucumber to measure 1 cup.

DICE THE CARROT

Peel and dice 1 carrot. Store with the yellow onion and 1 stalk of diced celery.

DICE THE CELERY

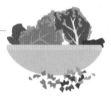

Dice 1 stalk of celery and store with the carrot and yellow onion. Dice 2 stalks of celery and store separately.

DICE THE YELLOW ONION

Dice enough yellow onion to measure ½ cup. Store with the carrot and 1 stalk of the celery.

CHOP THE KALE

Chop enough curly kale to measure 2 cups, removing any tough stems.

YIELD: 2 servings
PREP TIME: 10 minutes
COOK TIME: —

Breakfast
SALAD

4 cups arugula

4 soft-boiled eggs, peeled and halved √

4 slices turkey bacon, cooked √

1 red grapefruit, peeled and sectioned

½ Hass avocado, diced

¼ cup raw pecan halves

2 tablespoons extra-virgin olive oil

1 tablespoon lemon juice

1 tablespoon whole-grain mustard

Salt and pepper

1. Divide the arugula between two serving bowls. Top with the eggs, bacon, grapefruit, avocado, and pecans.

2. Make the dressing: In a small bowl, whisk together the oil, lemon juice, mustard, and salt and pepper to taste.

3. Drizzle the dressing over the salads and serve.

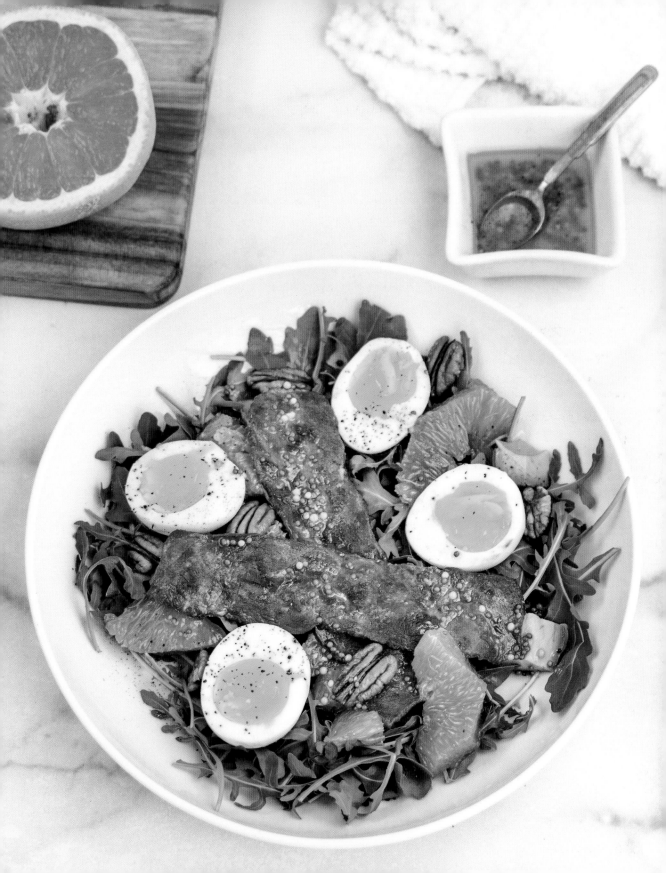

Pecan Pie
PROTEIN MUFFINS

YIELD: 8 muffins (2 per serving)
PREP TIME: 5 minutes
COOK TIME: 20 minutes

¾ cup raw pecan halves, divided

¼ cup (2 scoops) unflavored or vanilla-flavored protein powder

2 tablespoons hulled hemp seeds

1 teaspoon baking powder

½ teaspoon ground cinnamon

⅛ teaspoon fine sea salt

4 large eggs

½ cup unsweetened nondairy milk of choice

¼ cup coconut oil, melted

2 tablespoons molasses

1 teaspoon vanilla extract

NOTE:
These muffins freeze well, so you can freeze any leftovers that you do not plan on eating within the week for future use.

1. Preheat the oven to 350°F and spray 8 wells of a standard-size muffin tin with cooking spray.

2. Put ½ cup of the pecans in a blender and pulse to create a pecan flour.

3. In a large bowl, whisk together the pecan flour, protein powder, hemp seeds, baking powder, cinnamon, and salt.

4. Add the eggs, milk, oil, molasses, and vanilla and stir to combine. Fold in the remaining ¼ cup of pecans.

5. Pour the batter into the greased wells of the muffin tin, filling them about two-thirds full, and bake for 18 to 20 minutes, until a toothpick inserted in the center of a muffin comes out clean.

6. Remove from the oven, transfer the muffins to a cooling rack, and let cool. Serve, or store in the refrigerator for later in the week.

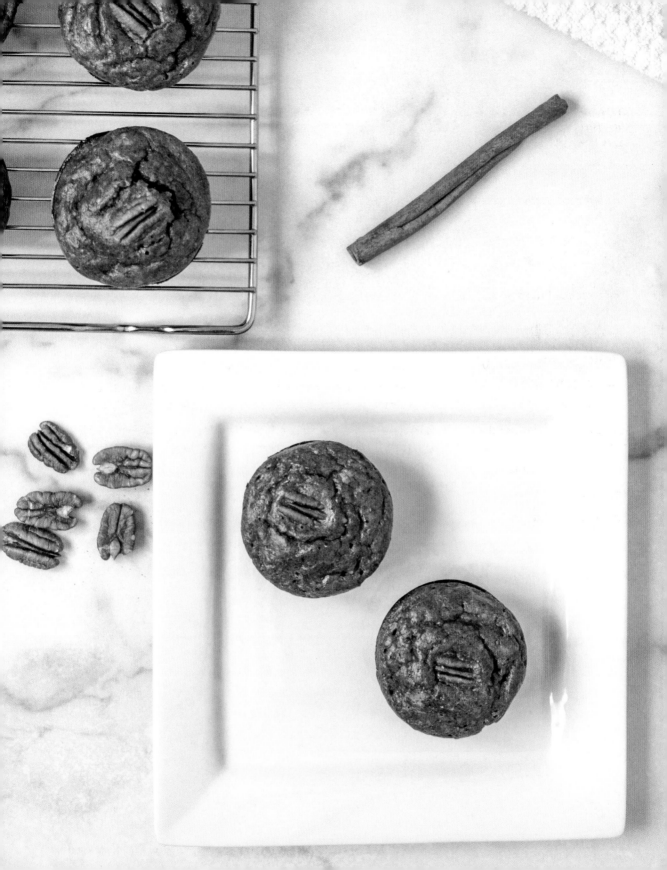

YIELD: 2 servings
PREP TIME: 10 minutes
COOK TIME: —

Mediterranean Chickpea
PASTA SALAD

2 tablespoons extra-virgin
olive oil

2 tablespoons lemon juice

1 tablespoon whole-grain
mustard

1 (5-ounce) can tuna packed
in water

2 cups arugula

1 cup cooked chickpea pasta √

1 cup diced cucumbers √

1 (15-ounce) can quartered
artichoke hearts (packed in
water), drained

1 (15-ounce) can white beans,
drained and rinsed

¼ cup thinly sliced red
onions √

¼ cup pitted Kalamata olives

¼ cup raw pecan halves

¼ cup sun-dried tomatoes

2 tablespoons capers, drained

Salt and pepper

1. In a large bowl, whisk together the oil, lemon juice, and mustard. Add the tuna and use a fork to break it up and combine it with the oil mixture.

2. Stir in the arugula, pasta, cucumbers, artichoke hearts, beans, onions, olives, pecans, sun-dried tomatoes, and capers. Season with salt and pepper to taste.

3. Serve, or store in the refrigerator for later in the week.

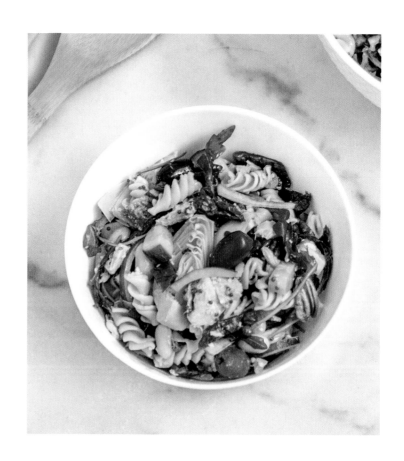

Fall
TUNA SALAD

YIELD: 2 servings
PREP TIME: 10 minutes
COOK TIME: —

1. Divide the arugula between two serving bowls.

2. In a medium bowl, whisk together the oil, lemon juice, and mustard. Add the tuna, apple, celery, pecans, and raisins and use a fork to break up the tuna and gently combine the ingredients. Season with salt and pepper to taste.

3. Top the arugula with the tuna salad and serve, or store the tuna salad for use later in the week.

4 cups arugula

2 tablespoons extra-virgin olive oil

2 tablespoons lemon juice

2 tablespoons whole-grain mustard

1 (5-ounce) can tuna packed in water

1 apple (any type), diced

2 stalks celery, diced √

½ cup raw pecan halves

¼ cup raisins

Salt and pepper

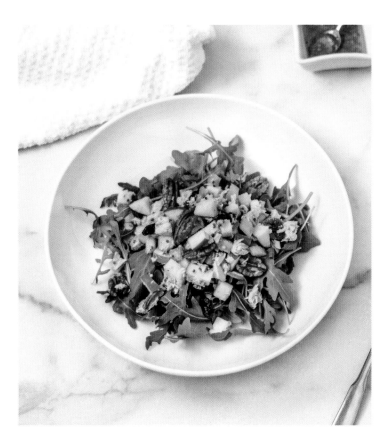

YIELD: 2 servings
PREP TIME: 5 minutes
COOK TIME: 15 minutes

Tuna Bolognese with
CHICKPEA PASTA

½ cup diced yellow onions √

1 carrot, diced √

1 stalk celery, diced √

1 tablespoon extra-virgin olive oil

1 (15-ounce) can tomato sauce

2 cloves garlic, minced √

1 teaspoon dried basil

2 tablespoons tomato paste

1 (5-ounce) can tuna packed in oil

2 cups chopped curly kale √

2 cups cooked chickpea pasta √

Salt and pepper

2 tablespoons grated Parmesan cheese, for topping (optional)

1. In a large skillet over medium-high heat, sauté the onions, carrot, and celery in the oil until softened, about 3 minutes.

2. Reduce the heat to low and add the tomato sauce, garlic, and basil. Cook, stirring, for 3 more minutes.

3. Stir in the tomato paste, then add the tuna, breaking it up with a fork. Add the kale and cook until softened, about 5 minutes.

4. Stir in the cooked pasta and heat until warmed through. Remove the pan from the heat and transfer the Bolognese mixture to serving plates. Season with salt and pepper to taste.

5. Top with the Parmesan cheese, if using, and serve, or store in the refrigerator for later in the week.

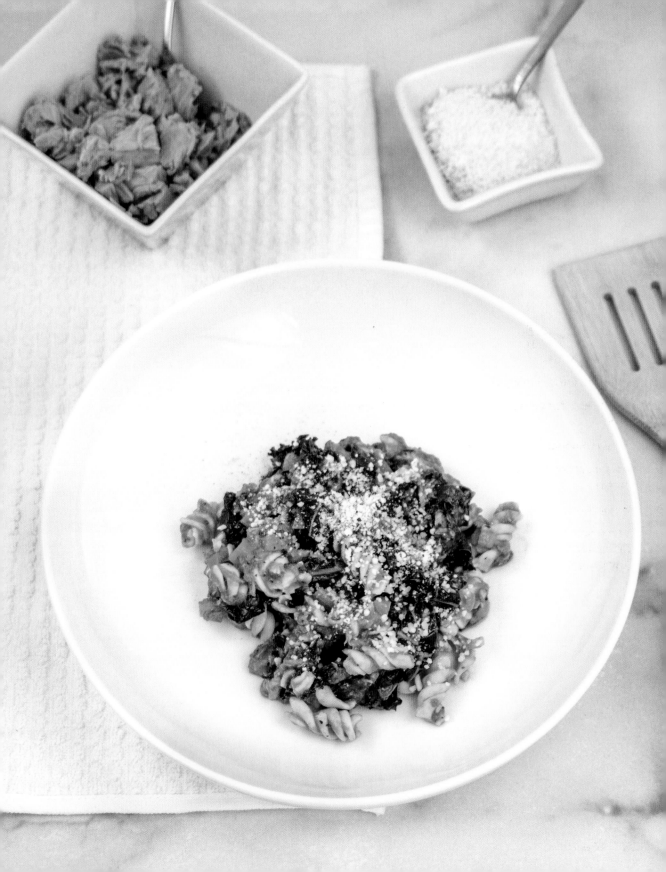

Seared Tuna with Arugula Pecan Pesto and MASHED CAULIFLOWER

YIELD: 2 servings
PREP TIME: 5 minutes
COOK TIME: 10 minutes

1 tablespoon extra-virgin olive oil

2 (4-ounce) tuna steaks

2 cups mashed cauliflower √

1 batch Arugula Pecan Pesto √

Salt and pepper

1. Heat the oil in a large skillet over medium-high heat. Add the tuna steaks and cook for 2 to 3 minutes on each side, until seared.

2. Warm the mashed cauliflower in the microwave or on the stovetop, then divide it between two serving plates.

3. Top the cauliflower with the seared tuna and spread the pesto over the tuna. Season with salt and pepper to taste. Serve, or store in the refrigerator for later in the week.

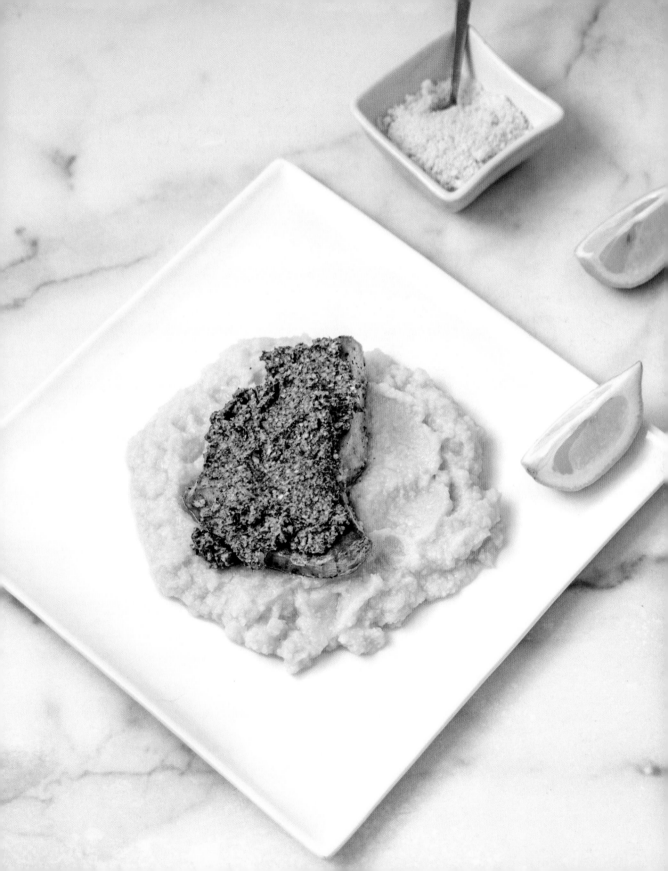

Week 14:

GROUND BEEF, WALNUTS, LENTILS, AND ROSEMARY

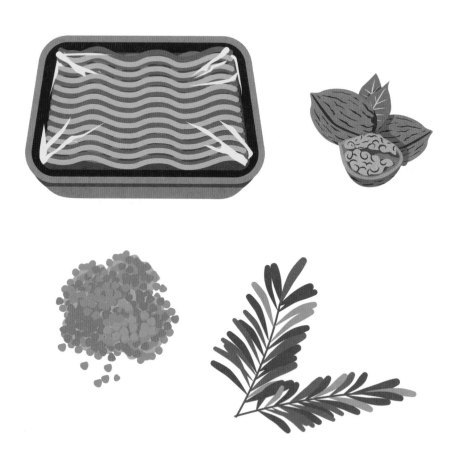

MENU

BREAKFAST	1	Warm Lentil Salad with Eggs
	2	Rosemary Breakfast Hash and Eggs
LUNCH	1	Lentil Beef Burger Wraps
	2	Meatball Salad
DINNER	1	Hidden Flax Meatballs with Rosemary Roasted Veggies
	2	Shepherd's Pie Bowls

FEATURED INGREDIENTS

 PROTEIN

This week's protein is ground beef, which is a good source of protein and nutrients. One serving provides nearly one-third of your daily vitamin B12 needs and 10 percent of your daily iron needs. If you want to eat less fat, you can look for 90 percent lean ground beef; otherwise, use 85 percent or 80 percent lean.

 FIBER

Lentils are this week's main source of fiber. One-half cup of cooked lentils provides 8 grams of fiber as well as 18 percent of the recommended daily value of iron, along with other important nutrients for PCOS, such as vitamin B6, magnesium, and zinc.

 FAT

This week's fat is walnuts, which are high in anti-inflammatory omega-3 fatty acids. They are also a good source of magnesium and B vitamins, both of which are beneficial for PCOS.

 PCOS POWER FOOD

This week's PCOS Power Food is rosemary. Rosemary is high in antioxidant and anti-inflammatory compounds, which may be beneficial for PCOS symptoms. Additionally, it may help lower blood sugar.

WEEKLY INGREDIENTS

FRESH PRODUCE

Acorn squash, 1 small

Apple (any type), 1

Brussels sprouts, 1 cup

Button mushrooms, whole or sliced, 8 ounces

Cauliflower, 1 head

Cherry tomatoes, 1 pint

Cucumbers, 2

Fennel, 1 bulb

Garlic, 8 cloves

Green lettuce leaves, 4

Kale, curly, 4 cups

Red bell pepper, 1

Romaine lettuce, 1 head

Spinach, 2 cups

Sweet potatoes, 2 medium

Yellow onions, 3

MEAT/SEAFOOD

Ground beef, 2½ pounds

EGGS/DAIRY/MILK

Eggs, 10 large

Full-fat plain Greek yogurt, 1 cup

Unsweetened nondairy milk of choice, 2 tablespoons

PANTRY

Apple cider vinegar, 1 tablespoon

Artichoke hearts, quartered, packed in water, 1 (15-ounce) can

Cooking spray (avocado or olive oil)

Dijon mustard, 1 tablespoon plus 1 teaspoon

Ground flaxseed, ¼ cup plus 2 tablespoons

Kalamata olives, pitted, ¼ cup

Lemon juice, 1 tablespoon

Lentils, dried, 2 cups

Olive oil, extra-virgin, ½ cup

Tamari, 1 tablespoon

Walnuts, raw, 1 cup

SEASONINGS

Dried oregano leaves, ½ teaspoon

Dried parsley, 2 teaspoons

Ground dried rosemary, 2 tablespoons plus ½ teaspoon

Red pepper flakes, 1 pinch

CUSTOMIZING THE PLAN

TO ADD MORE CARBS:

- Double the lentils.

- Have a piece of whole-grain toast with the Warm Lentil Salad and the Rosemary Breakfast Hash.

- Use whole-grain buns in place of the lettuce leaves in the Lentil Beef Burgers.

- Add ½ cup of cooked brown rice to the Meatball Salad and the Hidden Flax Meatballs.

- Double the sweet potatoes and omit the cauliflower in the mashed sweet potatoes for the Shepherd's Pie Bowls.

TO MAKE THIS WEEK DAIRY-FREE:

- Use a nondairy yogurt in place of the Greek yogurt.

PREP DAY

Today you will be cooking the lentils, making the Mashed Sweet Potato and Cauliflower and the Lentil Beef Burgers, and prepping some of the vegetables for the week.

Complete the following tasks and store each component in a separate container in the refrigerator for use later in the week.

COOK THE LENTILS

YIELD: 4 cups
PREP TIME: 5 minutes
COOK TIME: 25 minutes

Bring 2 cups dried lentils and 5 cups water to a boil in a large pot over medium-high heat. Cover, reduce the heat to a simmer, and cook until the lentils have softened, 20 to 25 minutes. Set aside 1 cup for the Lentil Beef Burgers and store the rest for use later in the week.

PEEL AND DICE THE SWEET POTATOES

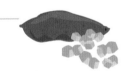

Peel and dice enough sweet potatoes to measure 2 cups. Set aside 1 cup for the Mashed Sweet Potato and Cauliflower and store the rest for use later in the week.

CHOP THE CAULIFLOWER

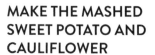

Roughly chop enough cauliflower to measure 2 cups. Set aside 1 cup for the Mashed Sweet Potato and Cauliflower and store the rest for use later in the week.

MAKE THE MASHED SWEET POTATO AND CAULIFLOWER

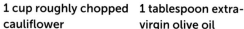

YIELD: 2 cups
PREP TIME: 10 minutes
COOK TIME: 10 minutes

1 cup roughly chopped cauliflower

1 cup peeled and diced sweet potatoes

1 cup water

2 tablespoons unsweetened nondairy milk of choice

1 tablespoon extra-virgin olive oil

1 clove garlic, minced

Salt and pepper

Put the cauliflower and sweet potatoes in a pot and pour in the water. Bring to a boil over medium-high heat. Once the sweet potatoes are tender, remove the pot from the heat and drain the water. Add the nondairy milk, olive oil, garlic, and salt and pepper to taste. Mash using a potato masher or an immersion blender until smooth.

DICE THE ONIONS

Dice enough yellow onions to measure 2¼ cups. Set aside ½ cup for the Lentil Beef Burgers and store the rest for use later in the week.

MINCE THE GARLIC

Peel and mince 8 cloves of garlic. Set aside 1 clove for the Mashed Sweet Potato and Cauliflower and 1 clove for the Lentil Beef Burgers and store the rest for use later in the week.

CHOP THE KALE

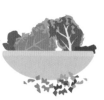

Chop enough curly kale to measure 4 cups, removing any tough stems.

CHOP THE SPINACH

Chop enough fresh spinach to measure 2 cups.

SLICE AND DICE THE CUCUMBER

Slice enough cucumber to measure 1 cup and dice enough cucumber to measure 1 cup. Store the sliced and diced cucumbers separately.

MAKE THE LENTIL BEEF BURGERS

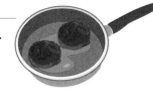

YIELD: 4 burgers
PREP TIME: 5 minutes
COOK TIME: 20 minutes

1 cup cooked lentils

½ cup diced yellow onions

½ cup raw walnuts

2 tablespoons ground flaxseed

1 clove garlic, minced

1 tablespoon tamari

1 teaspoon ground dried rosemary

1 large egg

⅛ teaspoon fine sea salt

⅛ teaspoon ground black pepper

8 ounces ground beef

1 tablespoon extra-virgin olive oil

1. Put the lentils, onions, walnuts, flaxseed, garlic, tamari, rosemary, egg, and salt and pepper in a food processor and pulse to combine.

2. Transfer the lentil mixture to a large bowl, add the ground beef, and use your hands to combine the ingredients. Form the mixture into 4 burger patties, about 3 inches in diameter and 1½ inches thick.

3. In a large skillet over medium-high heat, cook the burgers in the oil for 3 to 4 minutes per side for medium-done burgers, or to the desired doneness.

SLICE THE MUSHROOMS

Slice enough button mushrooms to measure 2 cups. (If you bought presliced mushrooms, skip this step.)

SLICE THE FENNEL

Trim and slice 1 bulb of fennel.

SLICE THE ACORN SQUASH

Halve a small acorn squash and use a spoon to scoop out the seeds. Cut the squash into ⅛-inch-thick slices.

HALVE THE BRUSSELS SPROUTS

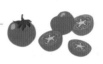

Trim and halve enough Brussels sprouts to measure 1 cup.

HALVE SOME OF THE TOMATOES

Halve 1 cup of cherry tomatoes.

Warm Lentil Salad
with EGGS

YIELD: 2 servings
PREP TIME: 5 minutes
COOK TIME: 13 minutes

½ cup diced yellow onions √

1 tablespoon extra-virgin olive oil

1 cup sliced button mushrooms √

1 clove garlic, minced √

1 teaspoon ground dried rosemary

1 cup cooked lentils √

2 cups chopped fresh spinach √

4 large eggs

1 tablespoon apple cider vinegar

1 teaspoon Dijon mustard

¼ cup chopped raw walnuts

Salt and pepper

1. In a large skillet over medium-high heat, sauté the onions in the oil until softened, about 3 minutes.

2. Add the mushrooms, garlic, and rosemary to the pan and cook, stirring, until the mushrooms have softened and are starting to brown, about 5 minutes.

3. Stir in the lentils and spinach and cook until the lentils are warmed through and the spinach is wilted, about 5 minutes. Stir the vinegar and mustard into the pan with the lentil salad and remove from the heat.

4. Meanwhile, spray a separate skillet with cooking spray and cook the eggs to your liking over medium-high heat.

5. Serve the warm lentil salad topped with the eggs and sprinkled with the chopped walnuts. Season with salt and pepper to taste. The salad can also be stored in the refrigerator for later in the week.

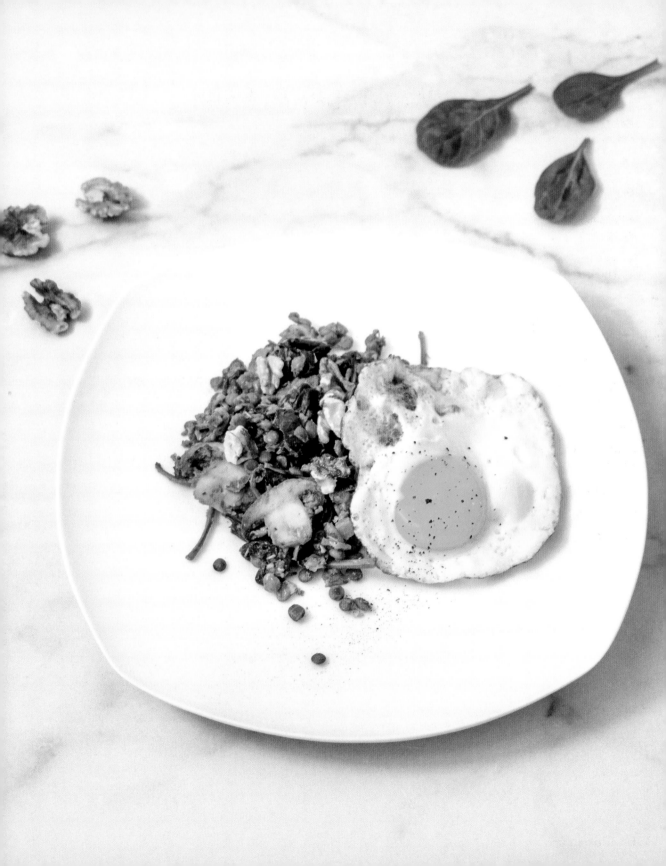

YIELD: 2 servings
PREP TIME: 5 minutes
COOK TIME: 28 minutes

Rosemary Breakfast
HASH and EGGS

½ cup diced yellow onions √

1 tablespoon extra-virgin olive oil

8 ounces ground beef

1 cup diced sweet potatoes √

1 clove garlic, minced √

1 teaspoon ground dried rosemary

2 cups chopped curly kale √

1 apple (any type), diced

4 large eggs

Pinch of red pepper flakes, for sprinkling

Salt and pepper

1. In a large skillet over medium-high heat, sauté the onions in the oil until softened, about 3 minutes.

2. Add the ground beef to the pan and cook, breaking up the meat with a spatula, until browned, 8 to 10 minutes.

3. Add the sweet potatoes, garlic, and rosemary to the pan and cook, stirring, until the sweet potatoes have softened, about 10 minutes.

4. Stir in the kale and apple and cook until the kale is wilted, about 5 minutes.

5. Meanwhile, spray a separate skillet with cooking spray and cook the eggs to your liking over medium-high heat.

6. Serve the warm hash topped with the eggs and sprinkled with the red pepper flakes. Season with salt and pepper to taste. The hash can also be stored in the refrigerator for later in the week.

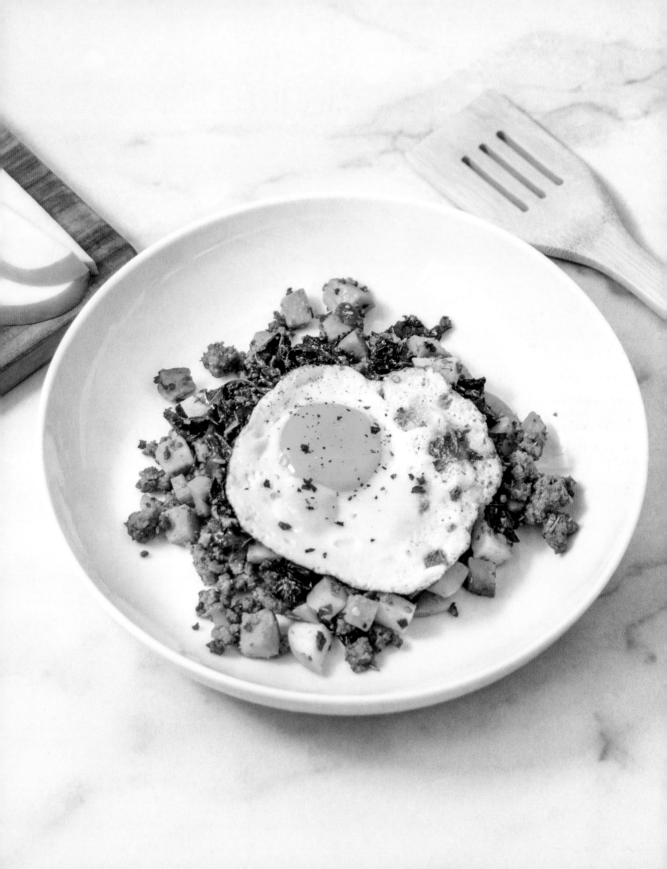

YIELD: 2 servings
PREP TIME: 5 minutes
COOK TIME: —

Lentil Beef
BURGER WRAPS

4 green lettuce leaves

4 Lentil Beef Burgers √

½ cup full-fat plain Greek yogurt

1 tablespoon Dijon mustard

Salt and pepper

1 cup sliced cucumbers √

1 cup cherry tomatoes

1. Place two lettuce leaves on each of two serving plates. Top each leaf with a burger.

2. Make the sauce: In a small bowl, whisk together the yogurt and mustard. Season with salt and pepper to taste.

3. Serve the burgers topped with the sliced cucumbers and cherry tomatoes and drizzled with the sauce.

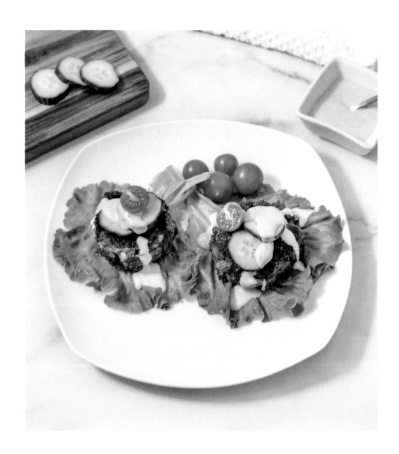

Meatball
SALAD

YIELD: 2 servings
PREP TIME: 5 minutes
COOK TIME: —

1. Divide the lettuce between two serving plates. Top with the meatballs.

2. Divide the lentils, tomatoes, cucumbers, red bell pepper, artichoke hearts, and olives between the two plates.

3. Make the dressing: In a small bowl, whisk together the yogurt, oil, lemon juice, oregano, rosemary, and salt and pepper to taste. Drizzle the dressing over the salads and serve.

4 cups chopped romaine lettuce

8 Hidden Flax Meatballs (page 252)

1 cup cooked lentils √

1 cup cherry tomatoes, halved √

1 cup diced cucumbers √

1 red bell pepper, sliced √

1 (15-ounce) can quartered artichoke hearts (packed in water), drained

¼ cup pitted Kalamata olives

½ cup full-fat plain Greek yogurt

2 tablespoons extra-virgin olive oil

1 tablespoon lemon juice

½ teaspoon dried oregano leaves

½ teaspoon ground dried rosemary

Salt and pepper

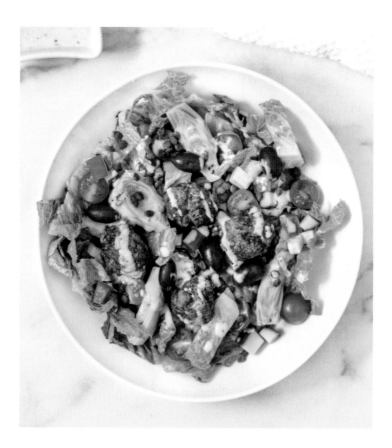

Hidden Flax Meatballs
with ROSEMARY ROASTED VEGGIES

YIELD: 16 meatballs (4 per serving)
PREP TIME: 10 minutes
COOK TIME: 20 minutes

1 pound ground beef

¼ cup ground flaxseed

1 large egg

¼ cup diced yellow onions √

2 cloves garlic, minced √

2 teaspoons ground dried rosemary, divided

1 teaspoon dried parsley

¼ teaspoon salt

⅛ teaspoon ground black pepper

1 bulb fennel, sliced √

1 cup Brussels sprouts, halved √

1 cup chopped cauliflower √

1 small acorn squash, cut into ⅛-inch-thick slices √

1 tablespoon extra-virgin olive oil

1. Preheat the oven to 400°F and line two sheet pans with parchment paper.

2. In a large bowl, use your hands to combine the ground beef, flaxseed, egg, onions, garlic, 1 teaspoon of the rosemary, and the parsley. Season with salt and pepper. Wet your hands, then roll the mixture into 16 balls, about 1½ inches in diameter, and place on one of the prepared pans.

3. Put the fennel, Brussels sprouts, cauliflower, and squash on the other prepared pan. Drizzle with the oil and sprinkle with the remaining teaspoon of rosemary. Season with salt and pepper.

4. Bake for 20 minutes, until the meatballs are browned with no pink remaining on the inside and the vegetables are golden brown.

5. Store half of the meatballs for use in the Meatball Salad (page 251). Serve the remaining meatballs with the veggies, or store in the refrigerator for later in the week.

NOTE:
These meatballs freeze well, so you can freeze any leftovers that you do not plan on eating within the week.

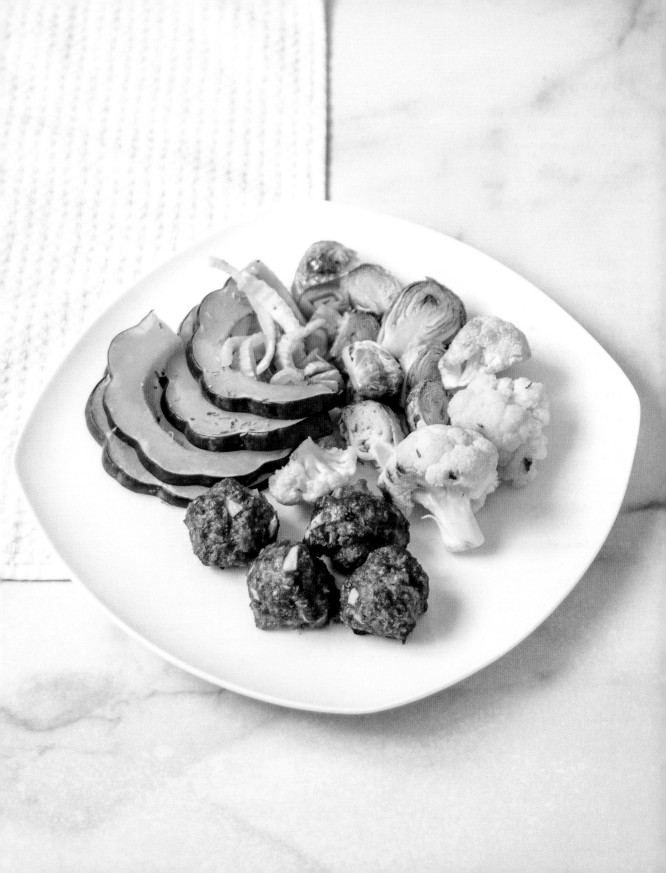

Shepherd's Pie
BOWLS

YIELD: 2 servings
PREP TIME: 5 minutes
COOK TIME: 20 minutes

½ cup diced yellow onions √

1 cup sliced button mushrooms √

1 tablespoon extra-virgin olive oil

8 ounces ground beef

1 cup cooked lentils √

2 cups chopped curly kale √

2 cloves garlic, minced √

¼ cup raw walnuts

1 teaspoon dried parsley

1 teaspoon ground dried rosemary

Salt and pepper

1 batch Mashed Sweet Potato and Cauliflower √

1. In a large skillet over medium-high heat, sauté the onions and mushrooms in the oil until softened, about 5 minutes.

2. Add the ground beef to the pan and cook, breaking up the meat with a spatula, until browned, 8 to 10 minutes.

3. Add the lentils, kale, garlic, walnuts, parsley, and rosemary to the pan and cook until the lentils are warmed through and the kale is wilted, about 5 minutes. Season with salt and pepper to taste.

4. Meanwhile, warm the Mashed Sweet Potato and Cauliflower in the microwave or on the stovetop.

5. Divide the beef and lentil mixture between two bowls. Top with the warm mash.

6. Serve, or store in the refrigerator for later in the week.

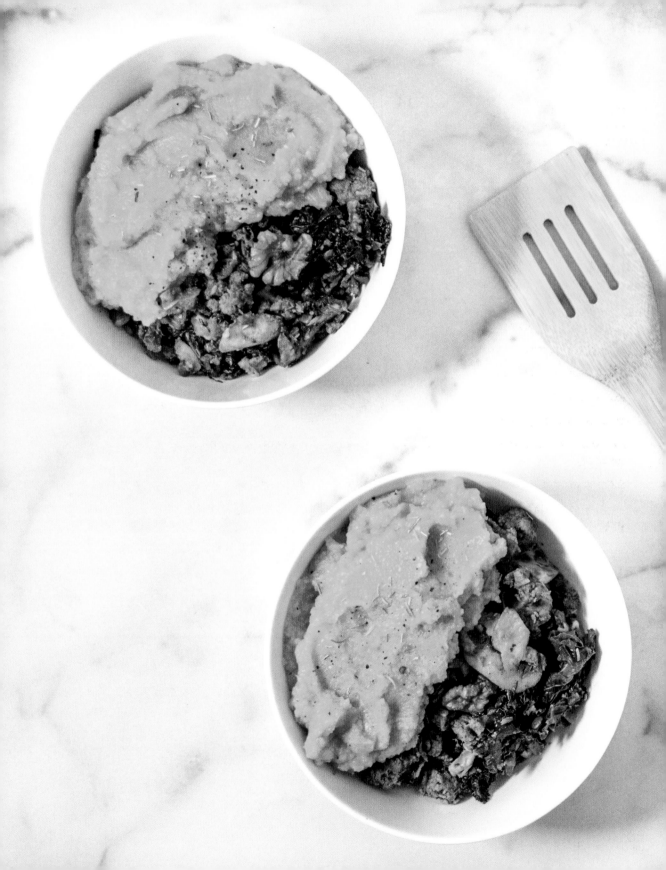

Week 15:

CHICKEN BREAST, SESAME SEEDS, BROCCOLI, AND CINNAMON

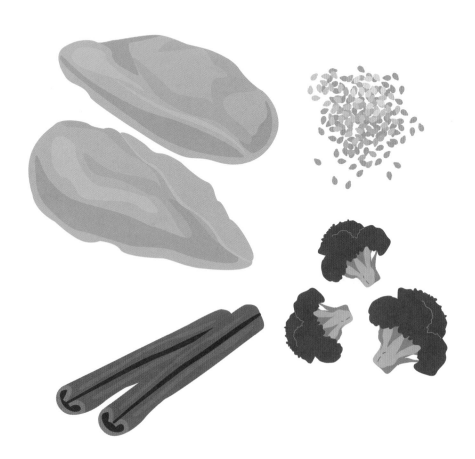

MENU

BREAKFAST	1	Toasted Sesame Protein Oats with Mandarins
	2	Cinnamon Roll Protein Muffins
LUNCH	1	Sesame Chicken Slaw
	2	White Chicken Chili
DINNER	1	Chicken Stir-Fry with Soba Noodles
	2	Sheet Pan Sesame-Crusted Chicken with Teriyaki Dipping Sauce

FEATURED INGREDIENTS

 ## PROTEIN

This week's protein is chicken breast, which is a lean source of protein. A 3.5-ounce serving has 115 calories and provides 21 grams of protein with less than 3 grams of fat. Chicken breast contains several nutrients beneficial for PCOS, including vitamins B6 and B12, iron, and magnesium.

 ## FIBER

Broccoli is this week's main source of fiber. One cup of chopped broccoli contains 2.4 grams of fiber and only 31 calories. It is high in antioxidant vitamin C and contains several plant compounds that may help the body metabolize estrogen.

 ## FAT

This week's fat is sesame seeds. In addition to healthy fats, sesame seeds provide about 1 gram of fiber per tablespoon. They contain lignans and phytosterols, which may help lower cholesterol and balance blood sugar. They are also a good source of magnesium, iron, and calcium.

 ## PCOS POWER FOOD

This week's PCOS Power Food is cinnamon. Cinnamon is high in antioxidants, and many studies show that it may help lower blood sugar and improve insulin sensitivity, making it a good choice for PCOS. It has anti-inflammatory properties as well.

WEEKLY INGREDIENTS

FRESH PRODUCE

Avocado, Hass, 1

Broccoli crowns, 2

Broccoli slaw, 1 (12-ounce) package

Carrots, 1 cup

Cilantro, 1 bunch

Garlic, 5 cloves

Ginger, 1 (2-inch) piece

Green onions, 6

Lime, 1

Mandarin oranges, 7

Poblano pepper, 1

Radishes, 4

Yellow onion, 1

FROZEN

Corn, ½ cup

MEAT/SEAFOOD

Chicken breasts, boneless, skinless,
2 pounds

EGGS/DAIRY/MILK

Eggs, 5 large

Unsweetened nondairy milk of choice,
2 cups

PANTRY

Avocado oil, 3 tablespoons

Baking powder, 1 teaspoon

Chia seeds, 2 tablespoons

Chicken bone broth, 1 cup plus
2 tablespoons

Coconut cream, ⅓ cup

Coconut oil, ¼ cup

Cooking spray (avocado or olive oil)

Dark (toasted) sesame oil, 2 teaspoons

Ground flaxseed, 2 tablespoons

Honey, 1 teaspoon

Lime juice, 1 tablespoon

Maple syrup, ¼ cup plus 1 tablespoon

Old-fashioned oats, 1¼ cups

Protein powder, ½ cup (4 scoops)

Rice vinegar, 2 tablespoons

Sesame seeds, ½ cup plus 1 tablespoon

Soba noodles, 4 ounces

Tamari, ½ cup

Vanilla extract, 2½ teaspoons

White beans, 1 (15-ounce) can

SEASONINGS

Ground cinnamon, 1 tablespoon

Ground cumin, 1 teaspoon

Red pepper flakes, ½ teaspoon plus
1 pinch

FALL

CUSTOMIZING THE PLAN

TO ADD MORE CARBS:

- Double the oats in the Toasted Sesame Protein Oats.

- Add cooked soba noodles to the Sesame Chicken Slaw.

- Serve the White Chicken Chili with cooked brown rice or tortilla chips.

- Double the soba noodles in the Chicken Stir-Fry.

- Serve the Sheet Pan Sesame-Crusted Chicken with cooked brown rice or soba noodles.

PREP DAY

Today you will be cooking some of the chicken and prepping some of the vegetables for the week. Also bake the Cinnamon Roll Protein Muffins (page 262) and make the Toasted Sesame Protein Oats (page 261).

Complete the following tasks and store each component in a separate container in the refrigerator for use later in the week.

COOK SOME OF THE CHICKEN

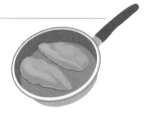

PREP TIME: 5 minutes
COOK TIME: 20 minutes

Heat 1 tablespoon avocado or extra-virgin olive oil in a large skillet over medium-high heat. Add 1 pound boneless, skinless chicken breasts and cook for 1 minute on each side. Season with salt and pepper. Cover and reduce the heat to low. After 10 minutes, remove the pan from the heat and let sit, covered, for another 10 minutes. The internal temperature should reach 165°F.

DICE THE YELLOW ONION

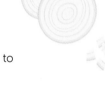

Dice enough yellow onion to measure ½ cup.

DICE THE POBLANO PEPPER

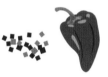

Dice 1 poblano pepper.

CHOP THE BROCCOLI CROWNS

Chop enough broccoli to measure 4 cups.

SLICE THE CARROTS

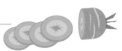

Peel and slice enough carrots to measure 1 cup.

SLICE THE RADISHES

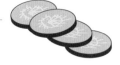

Thinly slice 4 radishes.

SLICE THE GREEN ONIONS

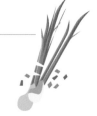

Thinly slice 6 green onions.

MINCE THE GARLIC

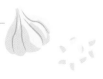

Peel and mince 5 cloves of garlic.

CHOP THE CILANTRO

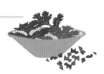

Finely chop enough fresh cilantro to measure ¼ cup.

Toasted Sesame
PROTEIN OATS with MANDARINS

YIELD: 2 servings
PREP TIME: 3 minutes
COOK TIME: 10 minutes

1. Put the oats, milk, chia seeds, and cinnamon in a small saucepan over medium heat and cook, stirring frequently, until the milk is absorbed, about 5 minutes. Remove from the heat and stir in the protein powder.

2. In a separate small saucepan over medium-high heat, combine the orange sections, maple syrup, and vanilla. Cook, stirring, until warmed through, about 5 minutes.

3. Meanwhile, toast the sesame seeds in a small dry skillet over medium heat, watching them closely so they don't burn, for 1 to 2 minutes, until golden brown.

4. Serve the oats topped with the oranges and toasted sesame seeds, or store in the refrigerator for later in the week.

¾ cup old-fashioned oats

1½ cups unsweetened nondairy milk of choice

2 tablespoons chia seeds

1 teaspoon ground cinnamon

¼ cup (2 scoops) unflavored protein powder

4 mandarin oranges, peeled, seeded, and sectioned

1 tablespoon maple syrup

1 teaspoon vanilla extract

1 tablespoon sesame seeds

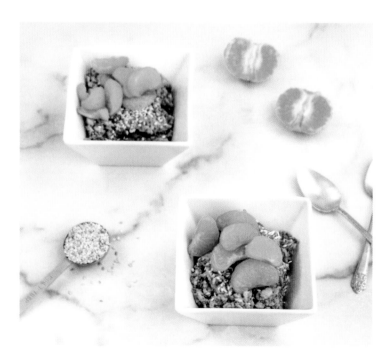

Cinnamon Roll
PROTEIN MUFFINS

YIELD: 6 muffins (2 per serving)
PREP TIME: 5 minutes
COOK TIME: 20 minutes

½ cup old-fashioned oats

¼ cup (2 scoops) unflavored or vanilla-flavored protein powder

2 tablespoons ground flaxseed

1 teaspoon baking powder

1 teaspoon ground cinnamon

⅛ teaspoon fine sea salt

4 large eggs

½ cup unsweetened nondairy milk of choice

¼ cup coconut oil, melted

2 tablespoons maple syrup, divided

1½ teaspoons vanilla extract, divided

⅓ cup coconut cream

NOTE:
These muffins freeze well, so you can freeze any leftovers that you do not plan on eating within the week.

1. Preheat the oven to 350°F and spray 6 wells of a standard-size muffin tin with cooking spray.

2. Put the oats in a blender and pulse to create an oat flour.

3. In a large bowl, whisk together the oat flour, protein powder, flaxseed, baking powder, cinnamon, and salt.

4. Add the eggs, milk, coconut oil, 1 tablespoon of the maple syrup, and 1 teaspoon of the vanilla and stir to combine.

5. Pour the batter into the prepared wells of the muffin tin, filling them about two-thirds full, and bake for 18 to 20 minutes, until a toothpick inserted in the center of a muffin comes out clean. Remove from the oven, transfer the muffins to a cooling rack, and let cool.

6. While the muffins are cooling, make the glaze: Put the coconut cream, the remaining tablespoon of maple syrup, and the remaining ½ teaspoon of vanilla in a small saucepan over medium-high heat. Cook, stirring, for 5 minutes. Remove from the heat and let thicken.

7. Dip the cooled muffins in the coconut glaze. Serve, or store in the refrigerator for later in the week.

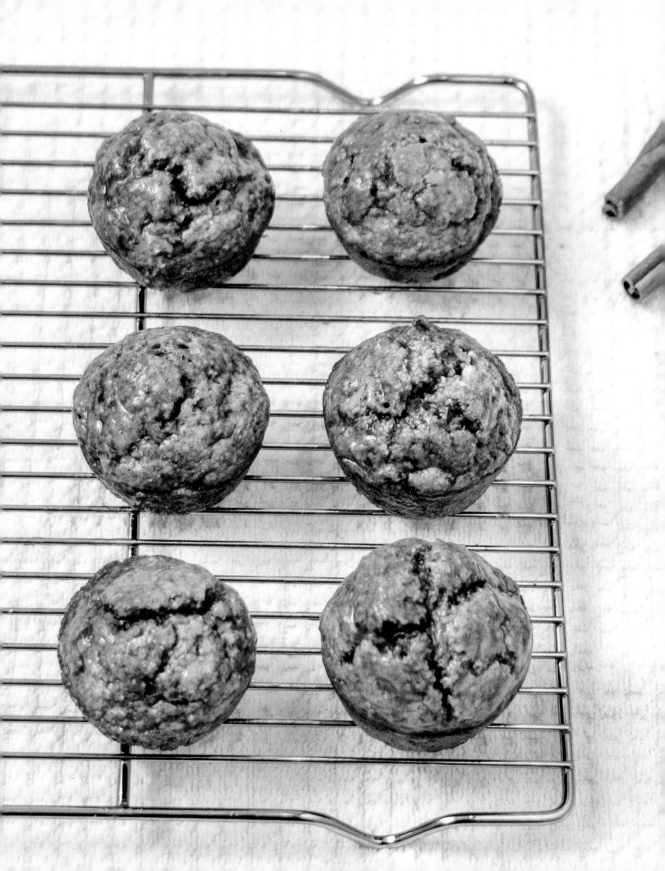

YIELD: 2 servings
PREP TIME: 5 minutes
COOK TIME: —

Sesame
CHICKEN SLAW

1 (12-ounce) package broccoli slaw (about 4 cups)

4 radishes, sliced √

4 green onions, thinly sliced √

1 mandarin orange, peeled, seeded, and sectioned

1 clove garlic, minced √

1 tablespoon minced ginger √

2 tablespoons sesame seeds

2 tablespoons tamari

1 tablespoon avocado oil

1 tablespoon rice vinegar

1 teaspoon dark (toasted) sesame oil

Half of the cooked chicken breast, sliced √

1. In a large bowl, combine the broccoli slaw, radishes, green onions, and orange sections.

2. Add the garlic, ginger, sesame seeds, tamari, avocado oil, rice vinegar, and sesame oil and toss to combine.

3. Serve topped with the sliced chicken, or store in the refrigerator for later in the week.

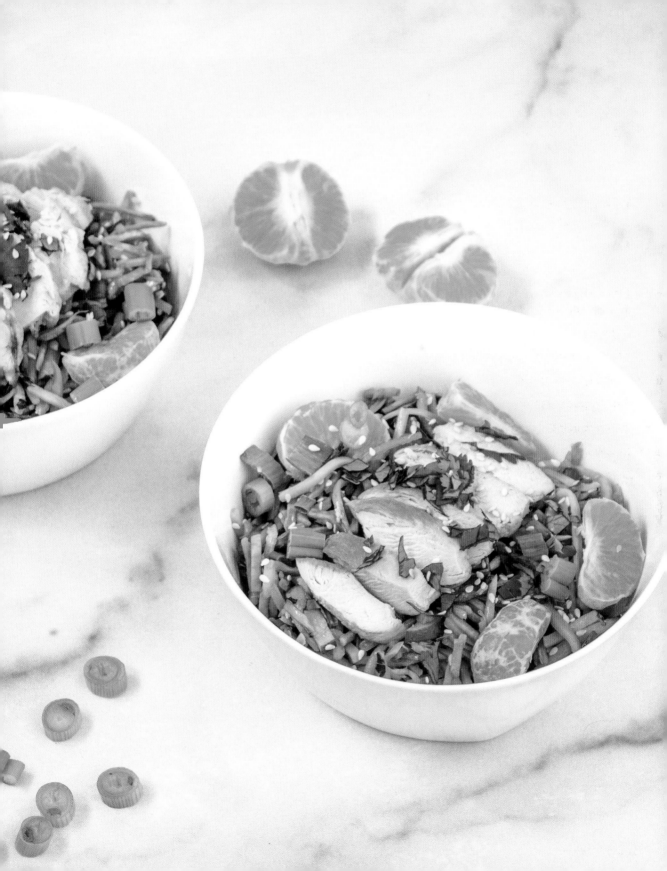

YIELD: 2 servings
PREP TIME: 5 minutes
COOK TIME: 20 minutes

White
CHICKEN CHILI

½ cup diced yellow onions √

1 poblano pepper, diced √

1 tablespoon avocado oil

1 cup chicken bone broth

1 (15-ounce) can white beans, drained and rinsed

½ cup frozen corn

1 clove garlic, minced √

1 teaspoon ground cumin

½ teaspoon ground cinnamon

Salt and pepper

Half of the cooked chicken breast √

¼ cup chopped fresh cilantro √

1 tablespoon lime juice

1. In a stockpot over medium-high heat, sauté the onions and poblano pepper in the oil until soft, about 5 minutes.

2. Add the broth, beans, corn, garlic, cumin, and cinnamon. Season with salt and pepper and stir to combine.

3. Shred the chicken and add it to the pot. Cover, reduce the heat to medium-low, and simmer for 10 to 15 minutes, until the chicken is warmed through.

4. Remove the pot from the heat and stir in the cilantro and lime juice. Serve, or store in the refrigerator for later in the week.

NOTE:
This chili freezes well, so you can freeze any leftovers that you do not plan on eating within the week.

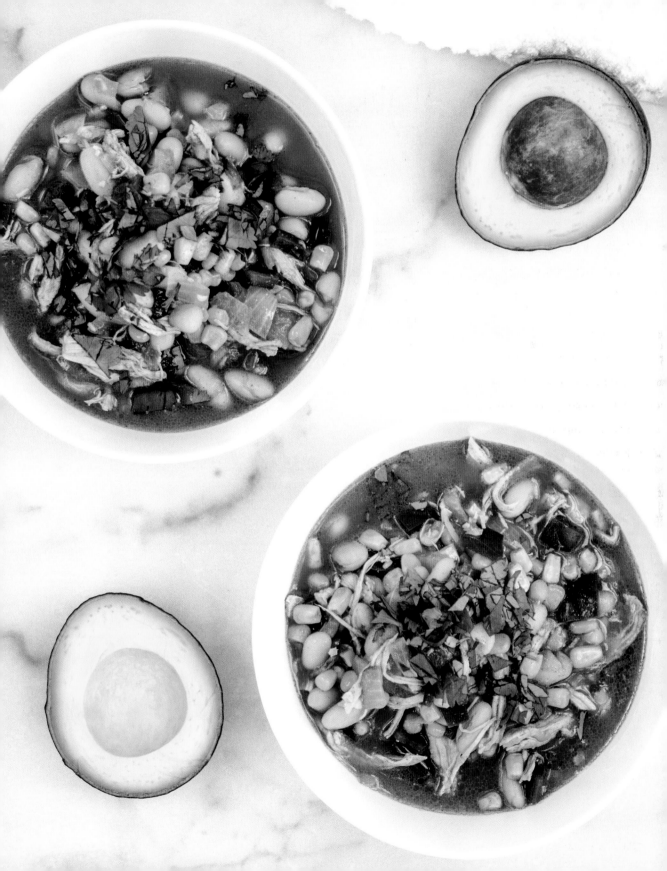

YIELD: 2 servings
PREP TIME: 10 minutes
COOK TIME: 20 minutes

Chicken Stir-Fry
with SOBA NOODLES

4 ounces soba noodles

1 tablespoon avocado oil

8 ounces boneless, skinless chicken breast

2 cups chopped broccoli √

1 tablespoon minced ginger √

2 cloves garlic, minced √

2 tablespoons chicken bone broth

1 tablespoon tamari

2 mandarin oranges, peeled, seeded, and sectioned

2 tablespoons sesame seeds

2 green onions, thinly sliced, for garnish √

Pinch of red pepper flakes, for garnish

1. Cook the soba noodles according to the package directions. Drain, then set aside.

2. Meanwhile, heat the oil in a large skillet. Cut the chicken into bite-sized pieces and add them to the pan. Cook until starting to brown and no longer pink inside, 5 to 7 minutes.

3. Add the broccoli, ginger, garlic, broth, and tamari to the skillet with the chicken. Cook, stirring, until the broccoli is crisp-tender, about 5 minutes.

4. Add the oranges and sesame seeds to the skillet and stir to combine. When the oranges are warmed through, remove the pan from the heat.

5. Divide the noodles between two serving plates and top with the chicken and vegetables. Garnish with the green onions and red pepper flakes and serve, or store in the refrigerator for later in the week.

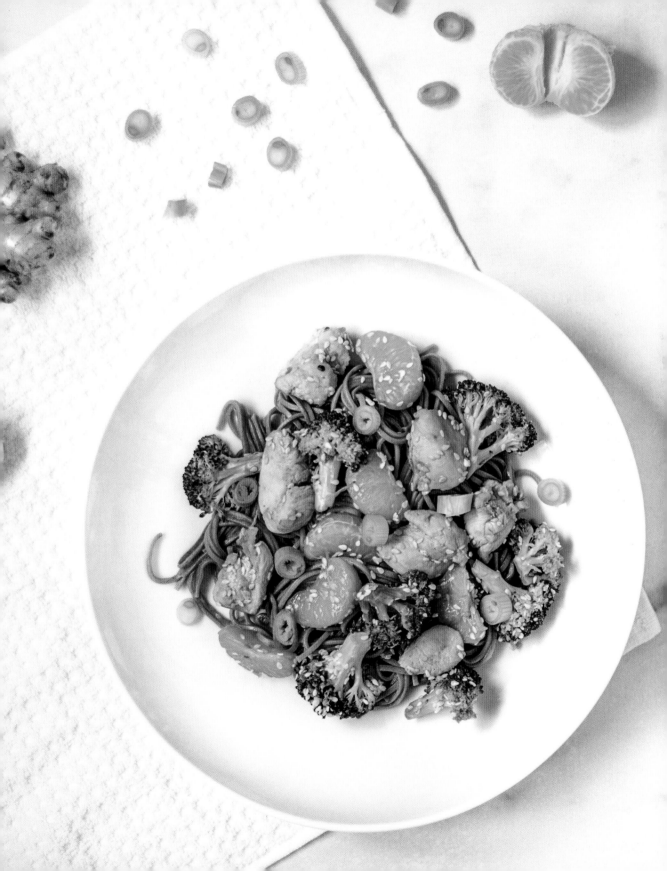

Sheet Pan Sesame-Crusted Chicken with
TERIYAKI DIPPING SAUCE

YIELD: 2 servings
PREP TIME: 5 minutes
COOK TIME: 25 minutes

1 large egg

¼ cup sesame seeds

8 ounces boneless, skinless chicken breast

Salt and pepper

2 cups chopped broccoli √

1 cup sliced carrots √

¼ cup tamari

1 tablespoon rice vinegar

1 teaspoon honey

1 teaspoon toasted sesame oil

1 tablespoon minced ginger √

1 clove garlic, minced √

½ teaspoon ground cinnamon

½ teaspoon red pepper flakes

1. Preheat the oven to 375°F. Line a sheet pan with parchment paper.

2. In a medium bowl, beat the egg. Put the sesame seeds on a plate.

3. Slice the chicken into thin strips. Dip each slice in the egg, then in the sesame seeds to coat, and place on the prepared pan. Season the coated chicken with salt and pepper.

4. Add the broccoli and carrots to the pan with the chicken. Bake for 25 minutes, or until golden brown and no longer pink in the center.

5. Meanwhile, make the dipping sauce: Put the remaining ingredients in a small saucepan and simmer over medium heat for 5 minutes. Strain out the solids.

6. Serve the chicken and vegetables with the dipping sauce on the side, or store in the refrigerator for later in the week.

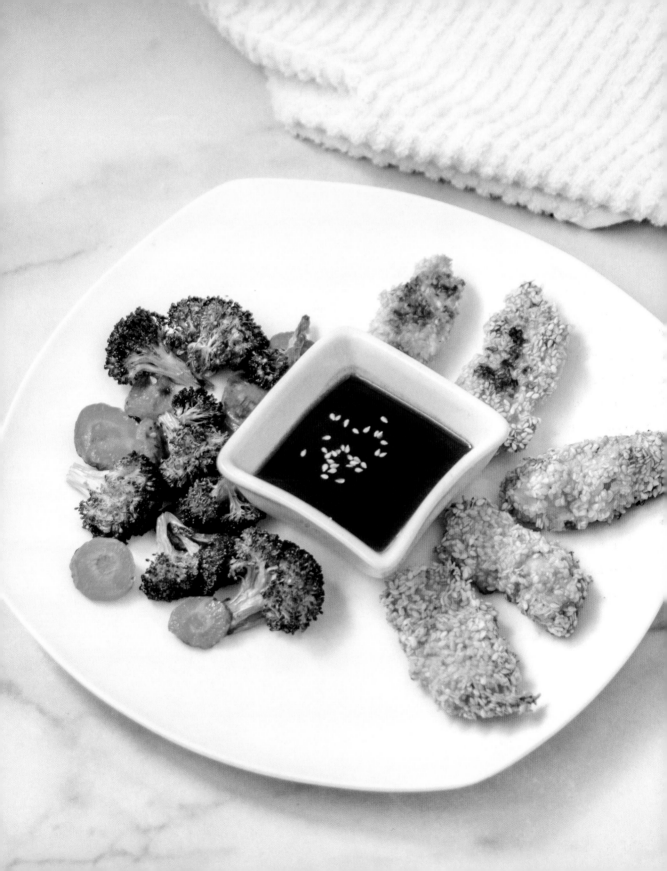

Week 16:

SAUSAGE, OLIVE OIL, PUMPKIN, AND BARLEY

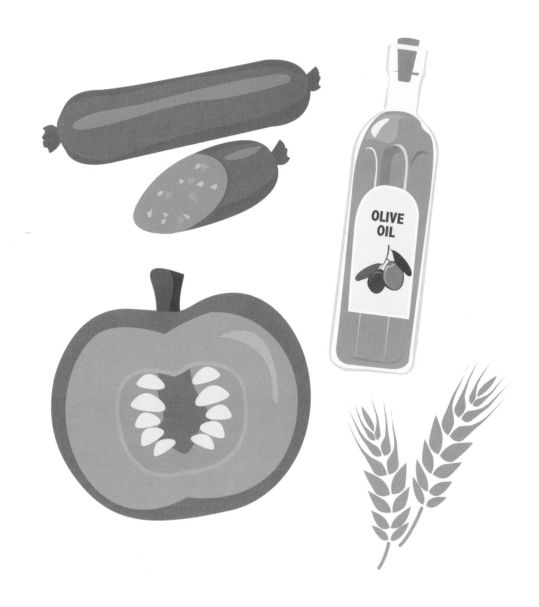

MENU

BREAKFAST	1	Pumpkin Spice Protein Oats
	2	Sausage Egg Muffins
LUNCH	1	Pumpkin, Sausage, and Leek Soup
	2	Sausage and Pepper Lunch Bowl
DINNER	1	Sausage and Barley Paella
	2	Sausage Barley Risotto

FEATURED INGREDIENTS

 ## PROTEIN

This week's protein is sausage, which is used in the recipes in bulk (uncased) form as well as Italian sausage links. While pork sausage is a higher-fat option, with 35 grams of fat per 4-ounce serving, it also provides 16 grams of protein and is an acceptable "once in a while" choice for PCOS. It is a good source of nutrients including vitamins B6 and B12 as well as iron. If you like, you can substitute a leaner turkey or chicken sausage in these recipes.

 ## FAT

This week's fat is olive oil, which is a staple of the anti-inflammatory Mediterranean diet. Extra-virgin olive oil is not only safe to cook with but adds a delicious flavor to almost any dish.

 ## FIBER

Pumpkin is this week's main source of fiber. One cup of pure pumpkin provides over 7 grams of fiber and only 83 calories, making it a smart lower-carb vegetable choice for PCOS. Pumpkin is high in many nutrients, including vitamins C, D, E, and K and several B vitamins. It is easy to add canned pumpkin to oats, muffins, smoothies, soups, and other dishes to increase the fiber content of a meal.

 ## PCOS POWER FOOD

This week's PCOS Power Food is barley. Barley has been shown in several studies to help lower blood sugar and insulin levels, making it an especially smart choice for PCOS. It is also high in fiber, and in particular soluble fiber, which may help lower cholesterol. Barley does contain gluten, so if you need to be gluten-free for medical reasons, swap out the barley in this week's recipes with another whole grain that is gluten-free, such as brown rice or quinoa.

WEEKLY INGREDIENTS

FRESH PRODUCE

Brussels sprouts, 1 cup

Button mushrooms, whole or sliced, 8 ounces

Carrot, 1

Celery, 1 stalk

Cherry tomatoes, 1 pint

Garlic, 9 cloves

Green bell peppers, 2

Kale, curly, 1 bunch

Leeks, 2

Parsley, curly or Italian, 1 bunch

Red bell pepper, 1

Red onion, 1

Shallots, 2 medium

Yellow onion, 1

FROZEN

Peas, ½ cup

MEAT/SEAFOOD

Bulk pork sausage, 12 ounces

Italian sausage links, mild or spicy, 1½ pounds

EGGS/DAIRY/MILK

Eggs, 8 large

Goat cheese or cheddar cheese, 2 ounces (optional, for the Sausage Egg Muffins)

Unsweetened nondairy milk of choice, ¾ cup plus 2 tablespoons

PANTRY

Artichoke hearts, quartered, packed in water, 1 (15-ounce) can

Barley, quick cooking, 1½ cups

Beef bone broth, 3½ cups

Cooking spray (avocado or olive oil)

Diced tomatoes, 1 (14-ounce) can

Ground flaxseed, 2 tablespoons

Hemp seeds, hulled, 2 tablespoons

Maple syrup, 1 tablespoon

Old-fashioned oats, ½ cup

Olive oil, extra-virgin, ½ cup

Pecans, raw, ¼ cup

Protein powder, unflavored, ¼ cup (2 scoops)

Pumpkin, 2 (15-ounce) cans

Vanilla extract, ½ teaspoon

SEASONINGS

Dried parsley, 1 teaspoon

Dried thyme, ½ teaspoon

Paprika, 1 teaspoon

Pumpkin pie spice, 2 teaspoons

Red pepper flakes, 1 pinch

CUSTOMIZING THE PLAN

TO ADD MORE CARBS:

- Double the barley.

- Double the oats in the Pumpkin Spice Protein Oats.

- Serve the Pumpkin, Sausage, and Leek Soup with a piece of whole-grain bread.

TO MAKE THIS WEEK DAIRY-FREE:

- Omit the cheese.

PREP DAY

Today you will be cooking the barley and sausage and prepping some of the vegetables for the week. Also make the Pumpkin Spice Protein Oats (page 278) and bake the Sausage Egg Muffins (page 280) so they are ready for the week.

Complete the following tasks and store each component in a separate container in the refrigerator for use later in the week.

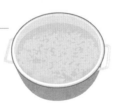

COOK THE BARLEY

YIELD: 3 cups
PREP TIME: 5 minutes
COOK TIME: 10 minutes

In a stockpot, cook 1½ cups quick-cooking barley in water according to the package directions.

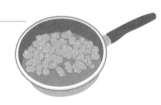

COOK THE BULK SAUSAGE

PREP TIME: 5 minutes
COOK TIME: 15 minutes

In a large skillet, cook 12 ounces bulk pork sausage until browned and cooked through, about 15 minutes. Season with salt and pepper to taste.

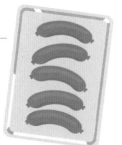

BAKE THE ITALIAN SAUSAGES

PREP TIME: 5 minutes
COOK TIME: 25 minutes

Preheat the oven to 400°F.
Place 1½ pounds Italian sausages on a sheet pan.
Bake for 20 to 25 minutes, until cooked through.
Cut into ½-inch slices.

ROAST THE BRUSSELS SPROUTS

PREP TIME: 5 minutes
COOK TIME: 25 minutes

Preheat the oven to 400°F. Trim and halve enough Brussels sprouts to measure 1 cup. Place on a sheet pan and drizzle with 1 tablespoon extra-virgin olive oil and 2 cloves minced garlic. Bake for 20 to 25 minutes, until crispy.

DICE THE SHALLOTS

Dice enough shallots to measure ½ cup.

MINCE THE GARLIC

Peel and mince 9 cloves of garlic. Set aside 2 cloves for the Brussels sprouts and store the rest for use later in the week.

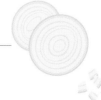

DICE THE YELLOW ONION

Dice enough yellow onion to measure 1 cup.

DICE THE RED ONION

Dice enough red onion to measure ½ cup.

DICE THE BELL PEPPERS

Dice enough green bell pepper to measure 1 cup and enough red bell pepper to measure ½ cup. Store the red pepper with half of the green pepper and store the rest of the green pepper separately.

DICE THE CELERY

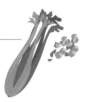

Dice 1 stalk of celery.

DICE THE CARROT

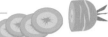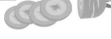

Peel and dice 1 carrot.

SLICE THE MUSHROOMS

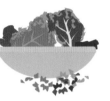

Thinly slice enough button mushrooms to measure 2 cups. (If you bought presliced mushrooms, skip this step.)

SLICE THE LEEKS

Cut off and discard the root ends and dark green parts of 2 leeks, then thinly slice the white and light green parts.

CHOP THE KALE

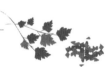

Chop enough curly kale to measure 2 cups, removing any tough stems.

HALVE THE CHERRY TOMATOES

Halve 1 pint of cherry tomatoes.

CHOP THE PARSLEY

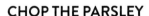

Finely chop enough fresh parsley to measure 1 cup.

YIELD: 2 servings
PREP TIME: 3 minutes
COOK TIME: 10 minutes

Pumpkin Spice
PROTEIN OATS

½ cup old-fashioned oats

¾ cup unsweetened nondairy milk of choice

1 cup canned pumpkin

2 tablespoons ground flaxseed

1 teaspoon pumpkin pie spice

Pinch of fine sea salt

¼ cup (2 scoops) unflavored protein powder

2 tablespoons hulled hemp seeds

1 tablespoon maple syrup

½ teaspoon vanilla extract

½ cup raw pecan halves, whole or chopped, for topping

1. Put the oats, milk, pumpkin, flaxseed, pumpkin pie spice, and salt in a small saucepan over medium heat and cook, stirring frequently, until the milk is absorbed, about 5 minutes.

2. Remove from the heat and stir in the protein powder, hemp seeds, maple syrup, and vanilla.

3. Top with the pecans and serve, or store in the refrigerator for later in the week.

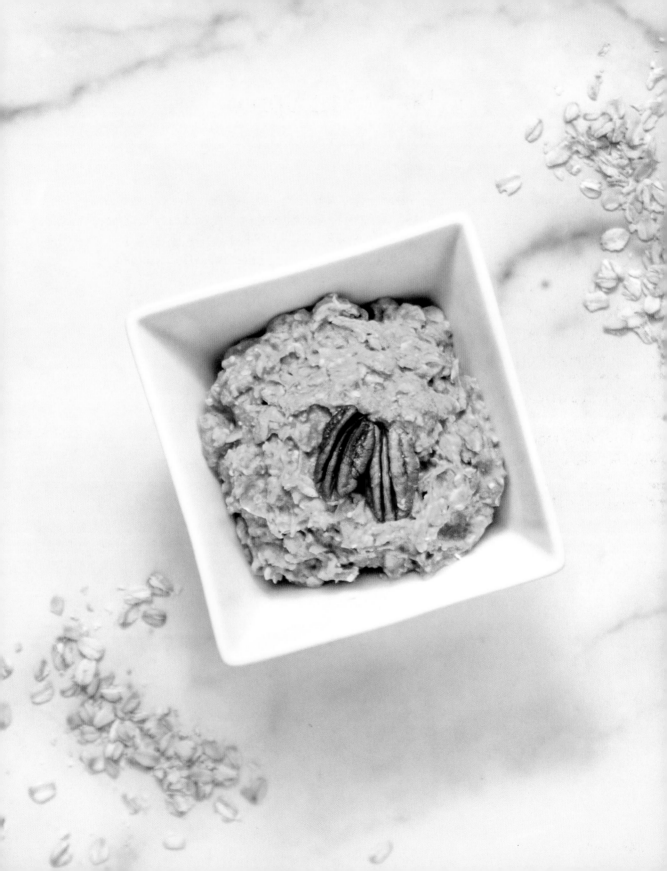

Sausage
EGG MUFFINS

YIELD: 8 muffins (2 per serving)
PREP TIME: 5 minutes
COOK TIME: 30 minutes

1 tablespoon extra-virgin olive oil

½ cup diced yellow onions √

½ cup diced green bell peppers √

½ cup diced red bell peppers √

One-third of the cooked pork sausage √

1 clove garlic, minced √

8 large eggs

2 tablespoons unsweetened nondairy milk of choice

¼ teaspoon salt

2 ounces goat cheese, crumbled, or cheddar cheese, shredded (optional)

1. Preheat the oven to 350°F and spray 8 wells of a standard-size muffin tin with cooking spray.

2. In a large skillet over medium-high heat, sauté the onions in the oil for 3 minutes, or until softened. Add the bell peppers and cook until slightly browned, about 5 minutes.

3. Add the sausage and garlic and cook, stirring, until warmed through, about 5 minutes.

4. Meanwhile, in a medium bowl, whisk the eggs with the milk and salt.

5. Distribute the sausage and pepper mixture evenly among the prepared wells of the muffin tin, filling them about two-thirds full, then pour in the egg mixture. Sprinkle the cheese over the tops of the muffins, if using.

6. Bake for 20 minutes, or until firm in the center. Remove from the oven and let cool in the pan. Serve, or store in the refrigerator for later in the week.

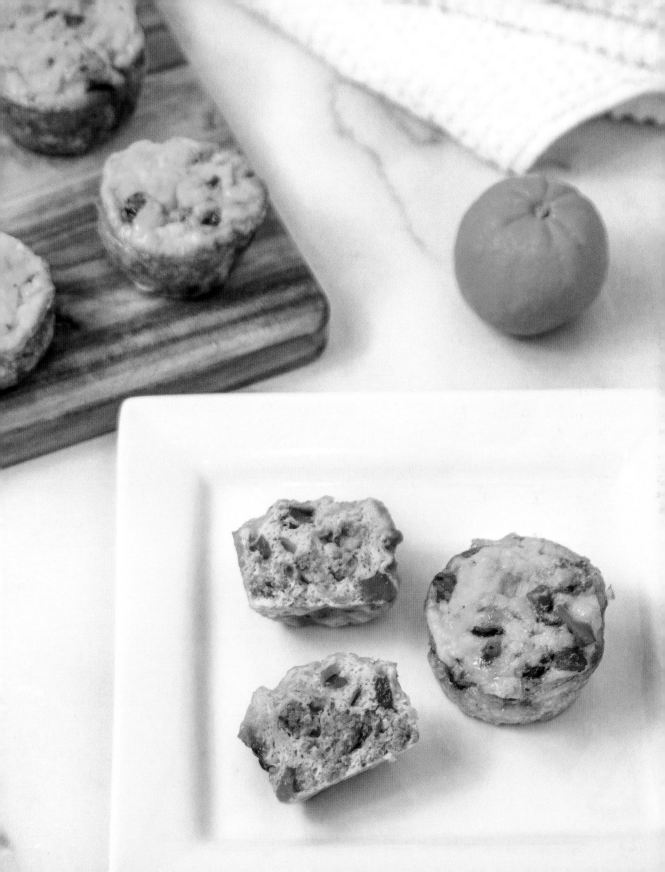

Pumpkin, Sausage, and LEEK SOUP

YIELD: 2 servings
PREP TIME: 5 minutes
COOK TIME: 10 minutes

2 leeks, sliced √

2 tablespoons extra-virgin olive oil

1 (15-ounce) can pumpkin

2 cups beef bone broth

2 cloves garlic, minced √

½ teaspoon dried thyme

Two-thirds of the cooked pork sausage √

Salt and pepper

1. In a stockpot over medium-high heat, sauté the leeks in the oil until soft, about 5 minutes.

2. Add the pumpkin, broth, garlic, and thyme and cook, stirring, until warmed through, about 5 minutes.

3. Stir in the cooked sausage and season with salt and pepper to taste. Serve, or store in the refrigerator for later in the week.

NOTE:
This soup freezes well, so you can freeze any leftovers that you do not plan on eating within the week.

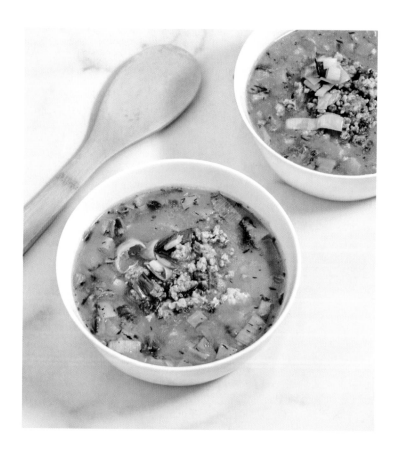

Sausage and Pepper
LUNCH BOWL

YIELD: 2 servings
PREP TIME: 10 minutes
COOK TIME: —

1. Arrange the barley, sausage, tomatoes, Brussels sprouts, bell peppers, and red onions in two serving bowls.

2. Make the dressing: In a small bowl, whisk together the oil, vinegar, parsley, and salt and pepper to taste. Drizzle the dressing over the bowls and serve.

1 cup cooked barley √

One-third of the cooked and sliced Italian sausage √

2 cups cherry tomatoes, halved √

1 cup Brussels sprouts, halved and roasted √

1 cup diced green bell peppers √

½ cup diced red onions √

2 tablespoons extra-virgin olive oil

1 tablespoon red wine vinegar

1 teaspoon dried parsley

Salt and pepper

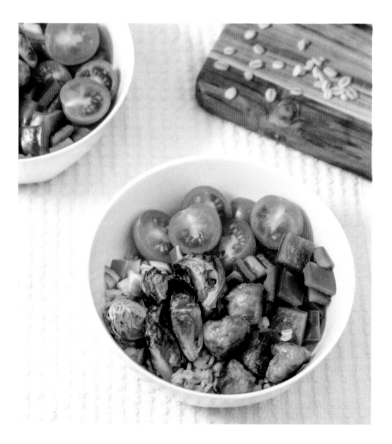

YIELD: 2 servings
PREP TIME: 5 minutes
COOK TIME: 20 minutes

Sausage and
BARLEY PAELLA

½ cup diced shallots √

2 tablespoons extra-virgin olive oil

½ cup beef bone broth

1 cup cooked barley √

2 cloves garlic, minced √

1 (15-ounce) can quartered artichoke hearts (packed in water), drained and rinsed

1 (14-ounce) can diced tomatoes

½ cup frozen peas

One-third of the cooked and sliced Italian sausage √

1 teaspoon paprika

½ cup finely chopped fresh parsley √

Salt and pepper

1. In a large skillet over medium-high heat, sauté the shallots in the oil until soft, about 5 minutes.

2. Add the broth, barley, and garlic and cook, stirring, until the barley is warmed through, about 5 minutes.

3. Add the artichoke hearts, tomatoes, peas, sausage, and paprika and cook, stirring, until warmed through, about 10 minutes.

4. Stir in the parsley and season with salt and pepper to taste. Serve, or store in the refrigerator for later in the week.

NOTE:
This dish freezes well, so you can freeze any leftovers that you do not plan on eating within the week.

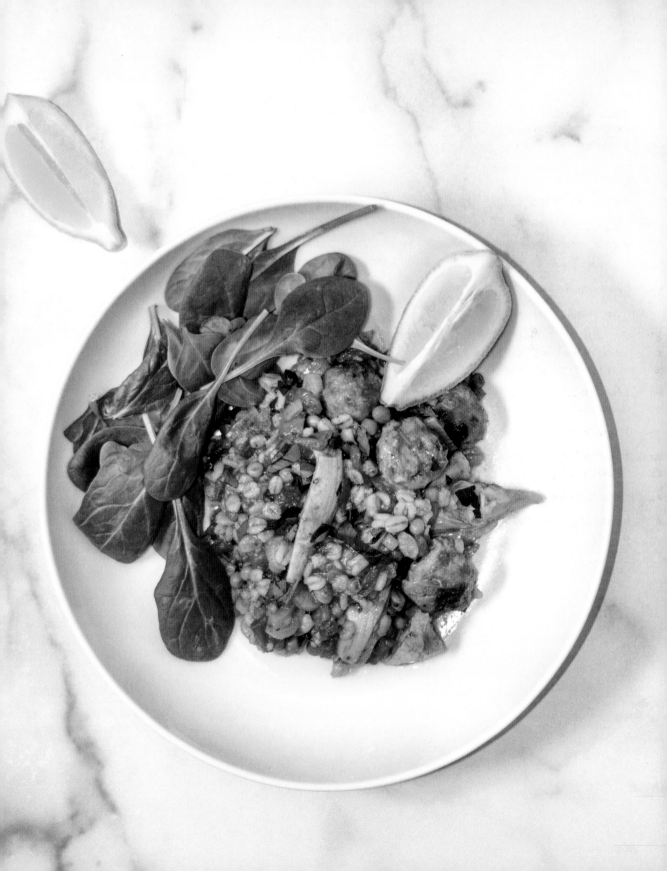

YIELD: 2 servings
PREP TIME: 5 minutes
COOK TIME: 20 minutes

Sausage Barley
RISOTTO

2 cups thinly sliced button mushrooms √

½ cup diced yellow onions √

1 carrot, peeled and diced √

1 stalk celery, diced √

2 tablespoons extra-virgin olive oil

1 cup beef bone broth

1 cup cooked barley √

2 cloves garlic, minced √

2 cups chopped curly kale √

One-third of the cooked and sliced Italian sausage √

½ cup finely chopped fresh parsley √

Pinch of red pepper flakes

Salt and pepper

1. In a large skillet over medium-high heat, sauté the mushrooms, onions, carrot, and celery in the oil until soft, about 5 minutes.

2. Add the broth, barley, and garlic and cook, stirring, until the barley is warmed through, about 5 minutes.

3. Add the kale and sausage and cook, stirring, until the sausage is warmed through and the kale is wilted, about 10 minutes.

4. Stir in the parsley, sprinkle with the red pepper flakes, and season with salt and pepper to taste. Serve, or store in the refrigerator for later in the week.

NOTE:
This dish freezes well, so you can freeze any leftovers that you do not plan on eating within the week.

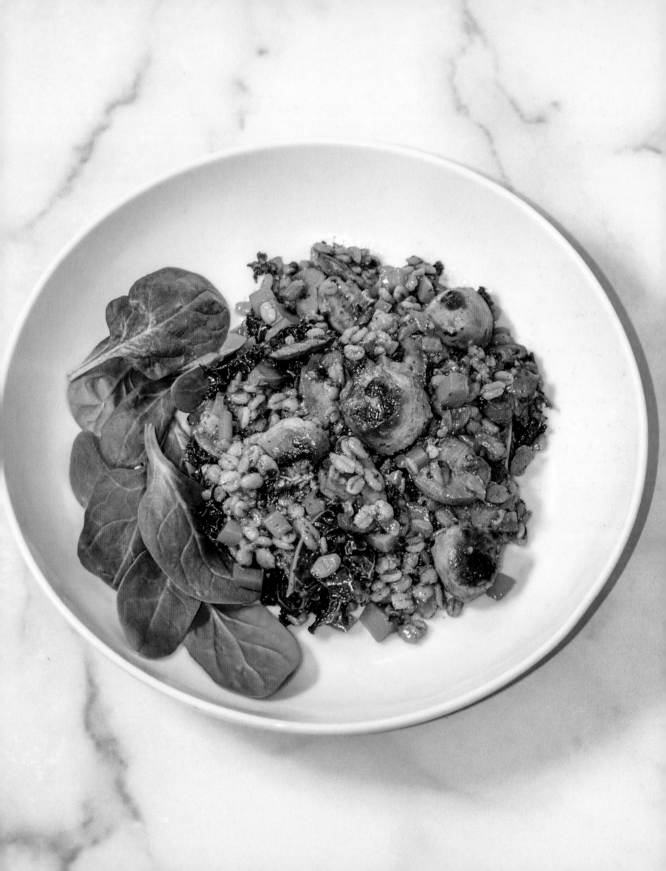

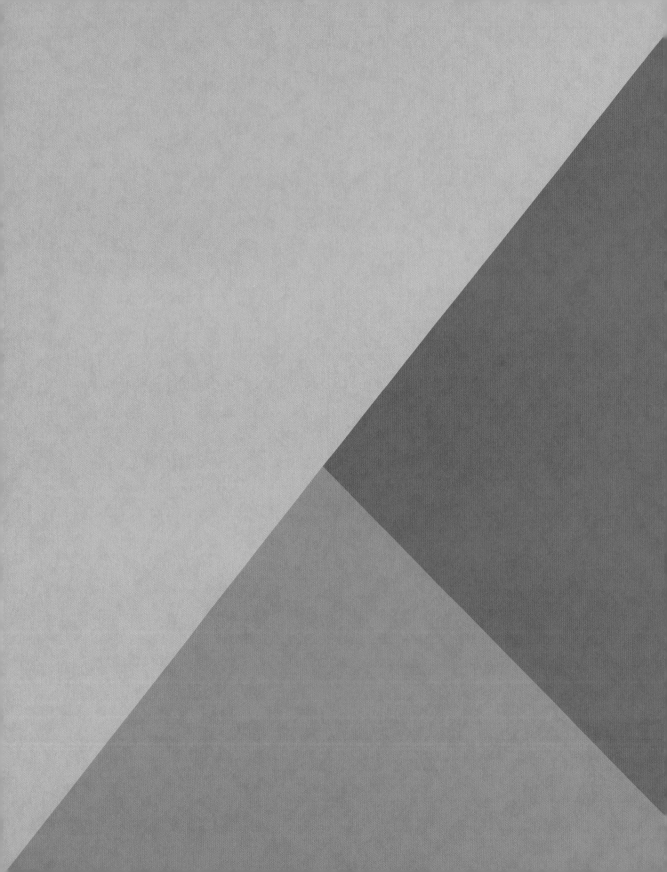

Part 2:

SUPPLE-MENTAL MENTAL RECIPES

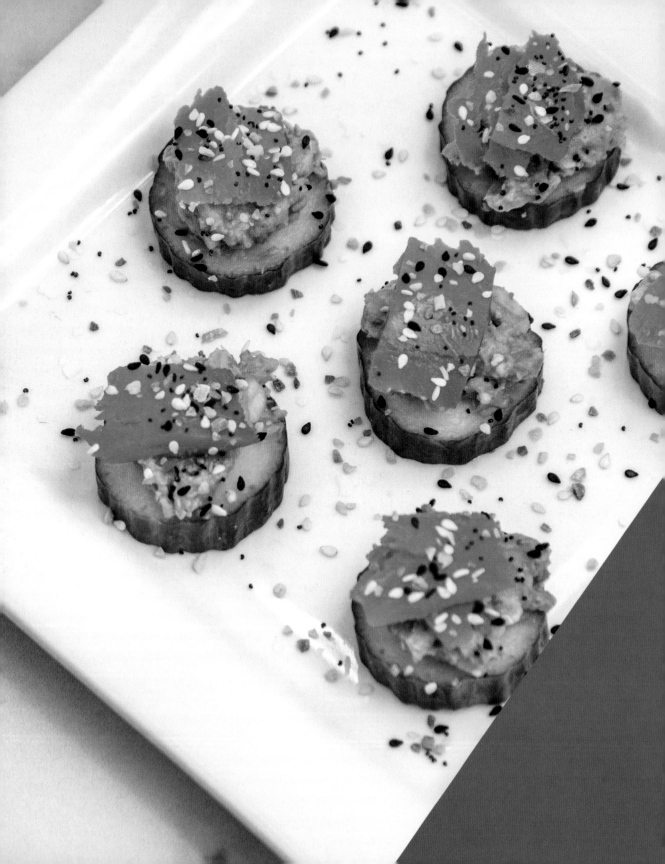

SNACKS

Oatmeal Cookie
PROTEIN BALLS

YIELD: 12 balls (2 per serving)
PREP TIME: 10 minutes, plus 1 hour to chill
COOK TIME: —

¾ **cup peanut butter**

½ **cup old-fashioned oats**

¼ **cup (2 scoops) collagen peptides or vanilla-flavored protein powder**

2 **tablespoons maple syrup**

1 **teaspoon ground cinnamon**

1 **teaspoon vanilla extract**

2 **tablespoons raisins or dark chocolate chips**

1. In a large bowl, combine the peanut butter, oats, collagen, cinnamon, and vanilla. Fold in the raisins.

2. Using your hands, roll the mixture into 12 balls, about 1 inch in diameter. Place the balls on a sheet pan.

3. Chill the balls for at least 1 hour before eating. Store in the refrigerator for up to 1 week.

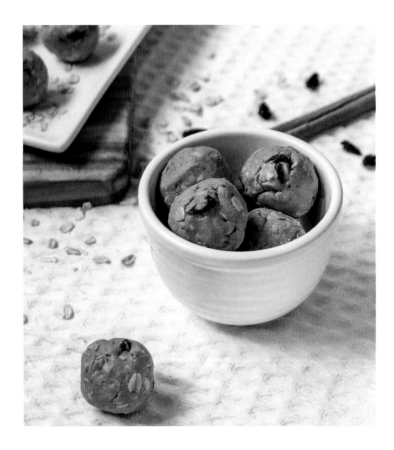

Instant
SUSHI

YIELD: 4 pieces (2 per serving)
PREP TIME: 5 minutes
COOK TIME: —

1. Slice the cucumbers into thin sticks. Thinly slice the avocado.

2. Layer the cucumbers, avocado slices, and smoked salmon on one half of each nori sheet. Roll the nori around the filling.

3. Serve immediately with the tamari, or store in the refrigerator for up to 3 days.

2 small cucumbers

½ Hass avocado

4 ounces smoked salmon

4 sheets sushi nori (dried seaweed sheets)

Tamari, for dipping

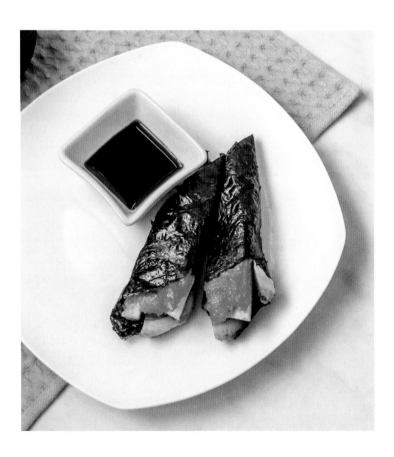

Coconut Matcha
PROTEIN BALLS

YIELD: 15 balls (2 per serving)
PREP TIME: 10 minutes, plus
1 hour to chill
COOK TIME: —

½ cup cashew butter

½ cup coconut flour

¼ cup coconut oil, melted

¼ cup coconut sugar

¼ cup (2 scoops) collagen peptides or vanilla-flavored protein powder

1 teaspoon matcha powder

1 teaspoon vanilla extract

1 cup unsweetened shredded coconut, divided

1. In a large bowl, combine the cashew butter, coconut flour, coconut oil, coconut sugar, collagen, matcha, vanilla, and ½ cup of the shredded coconut.

2. Using your hands, roll the mixture into 15 balls, about 1 inch in diameter. Roll each ball in the remaining ½ cup of shredded coconut. Place the balls on a sheet pan.

3. Chill the balls for at least 1 hour before eating. Store in the refrigerator for up to 1 week.

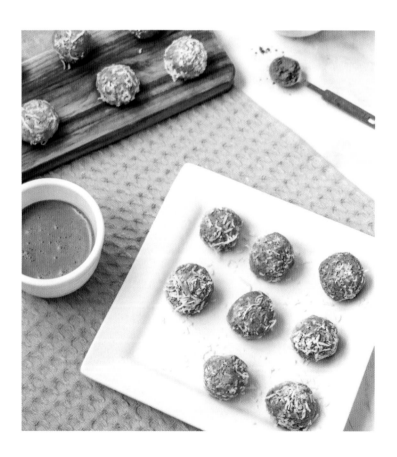

Green Goddess
HUMMUS

YIELD: 8 servings (about ½ cup per serving)
PREP TIME: 5 minutes, plus 30 minutes to soak cashews and 1 hour to chill
COOK TIME: —

1. Soak the cashews in 1 cup of water for 30 minutes. Drain.

2. Put the drained cashews in a food processor. Add the remaining ingredients and pulse until a smooth paste forms.

3. Cover the hummus and chill for at least 1 hour before serving. Serve with the sliced raw vegetables of your choice.

½ cup cashews

1½ cups full-fat plain Greek yogurt or nondairy yogurt

1 (15-ounce) can chickpeas or white beans, drained and rinsed

½ cup fresh parsley

¼ cup fresh basil leaves

¼ cup lemon juice

1 tablespoon extra-virgin olive oil

1 tablespoon tahini

1 clove garlic, roughly chopped

¼ teaspoon fine sea salt

Sliced cucumbers, bell peppers, or other vegetables of choice, or whole-grain crackers, for serving

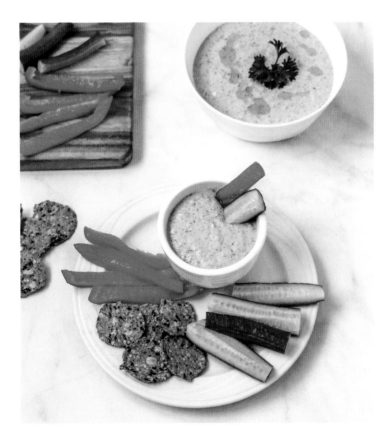

Apple Nachos with
SEED-NOLA

YIELD: 2 servings, plus 1 cup leftover seed-nola
PREP TIME: 10 minutes
COOK TIME: 20 minutes

FOR THE SEED-NOLA
(makes about 1½ cups):

½ cup unsweetened shredded coconut

½ cup pumpkin seeds

½ cup shelled sunflower seeds

1 tablespoon chia seeds

1 tablespoon ground flaxseed

1 tablespoon maple syrup

1 teaspoon ground cinnamon

¼ teaspoon fine sea salt

2 apples (any type)

2 tablespoons dark chocolate chips or chunks

1 tablespoon coconut oil

¼ cup full-fat plain Greek yogurt or nondairy yogurt

2 tablespoons dried cranberries

1. Preheat the oven to 325°F and line a sheet pan with parchment paper.

2. Make the seed-nola: In a large bowl, combine the coconut, pumpkin seeds, sunflower seeds, chia seeds, flaxseed, maple syrup, cinnamon, and salt.

3. Spread the seed mixture on the lined pan and bake, checking frequently, until golden brown and fragrant, about 20 minutes. Remove from the oven and let cool.

4. While the seed mixture is cooling, make the "chips": Thinly slice the apples and place them on a plate.

5. Put the chocolate and coconut oil in a small microwave-safe bowl and microwave for 30 seconds at a time, stirring after each increment, until melted.

6. Sprinkle ½ cup of the seed-nola over the sliced apples. Drizzle with the chocolate sauce and yogurt and top with the dried cranberries.

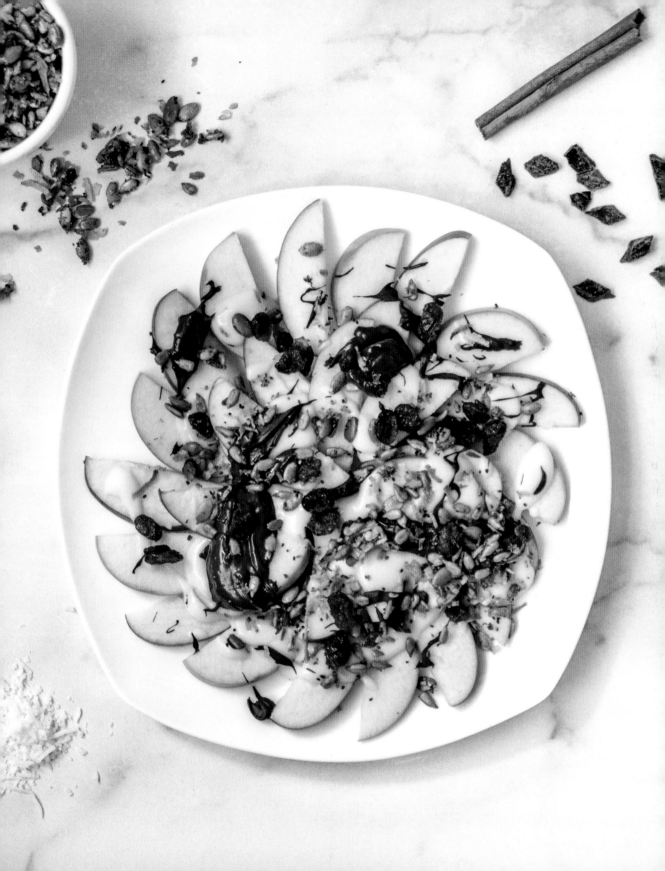

Avocado
PROTEIN TOAST

YIELD: 2 servings
PREP TIME: 5 minutes
COOK TIME: —

2 slices whole-grain bread

1 Hass avocado, peeled and pitted

4 ounces firm or extra-firm tofu

1 tablespoon lemon juice

½ teaspoon garlic powder

⅛ teaspoon fine sea salt

1 tablespoon hulled hemp seeds

2 teaspoons sesame seeds

½ teaspoon red pepper flakes

1. Toast the bread.

2. Meanwhile, in a medium bowl, mash the avocado with the tofu. Stir in the lemon juice, garlic powder, and salt.

3. Spread the mashed avocado mixture on the toast and sprinkle with the hemp seeds, sesame seeds, and red pepper flakes.

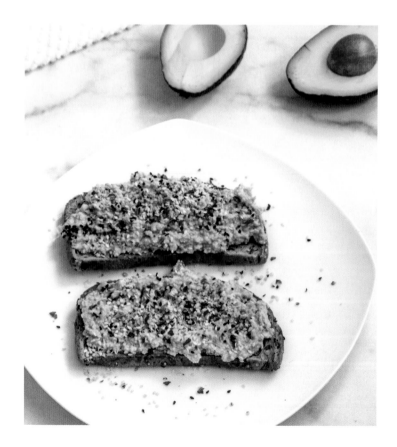

Smoked Salmon
CUCUMBER BITES

YIELD: 2 servings
PREP TIME: 5 minutes
COOK TIME: —

1. Slice the cucumber into 12 rounds, about ¼ inch thick.

2. In a small bowl, mash the avocado with the lemon juice. Spread the mashed avocado on the cucumber slices.

3. Cut the smoked salmon into 1-inch pieces and place on top of the avocado. Sprinkle with the everything bagel seasoning.

4. Serve, or store in the refrigerator for up to 3 days.

1 medium cucumber

1 Hass avocado, peeled and pitted

2 teaspoons lemon juice

4 ounces smoked salmon

1 tablespoon everything bagel seasoning, or 1 tablespoon sesame seeds plus ⅛ teaspoon fine sea salt

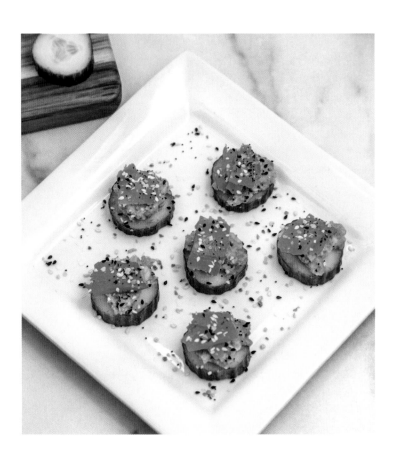

Anti-Inflammatory
TRAIL MIX

YIELD: 1¾ cups (¼ cup per serving)
PREP TIME: 5 minutes
COOK TIME: 10 minutes

½ **cup raw almonds**

½ **cup raw walnuts**

½ **cup dried cherries**

¼ **cup dark chocolate chunks**

1. Preheat the oven to 200°F.

2. Place the almonds and walnuts on a sheet pan and bake for 10 minutes, or until fragrant. Remove from the oven and let cool completely.

3. Stir the dried cherries and chocolate chunks into the cooled nuts.

4. Store in an airtight container for up to 2 weeks.

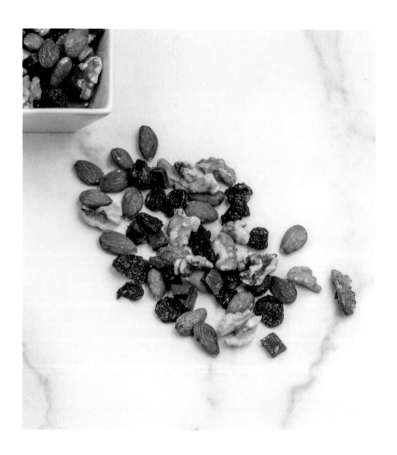

Chocolate
HUMMUS

YIELD: 8 servings (about ¼ cup per serving)
PREP TIME: 5 minutes, plus 1 hour to chill
COOK TIME: —

1. Put the black beans, milk, cacao powder, maple syrup, and collagen in a food processor and process until smooth. Transfer the hummus to a bowl, cover, and chill for at least 1 hour before serving.

2. Serve with sliced fruit for dipping.

1 (15-ounce) can black beans, drained and rinsed

¼ cup unsweetened nondairy milk of choice

2 tablespoons cacao powder or cocoa powder

2 tablespoons maple syrup

2 tablespoons (1 scoop) collagen peptides or chocolate-flavored protein powder

Sliced apples, strawberries, or other fruit of choice, for dipping

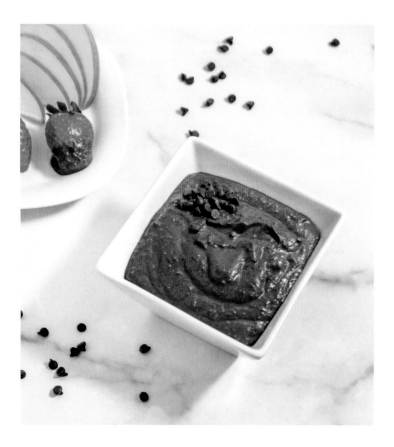

YIELD: 15 balls (2 per serving)
PREP TIME: 10 minutes, plus
1 hour to chill
COOK TIME: —

Pumpkin Cashew
PROTEIN BALLS

½ cup cashew butter

½ cup canned pumpkin

½ cup coconut flour

¼ cup (2 scoops) collagen
peptides or vanilla-flavored
protein powder

2 tablespoons maple syrup

1 teaspoon pumpkin pie spice

¼ cup hulled hemp seeds or
unsweetened coconut flakes,
for rolling (optional)

1. In a large bowl, combine all the ingredients except the hemp seeds, if using.

2. Using your hands, roll the mixture into 15 balls, about 1 inch in diameter. Roll each ball in the hemp seeds, if desired. Place the balls on a sheet pan.

3. Chill the balls for at least 1 hour before eating. Store in the refrigerator for up to 1 week.

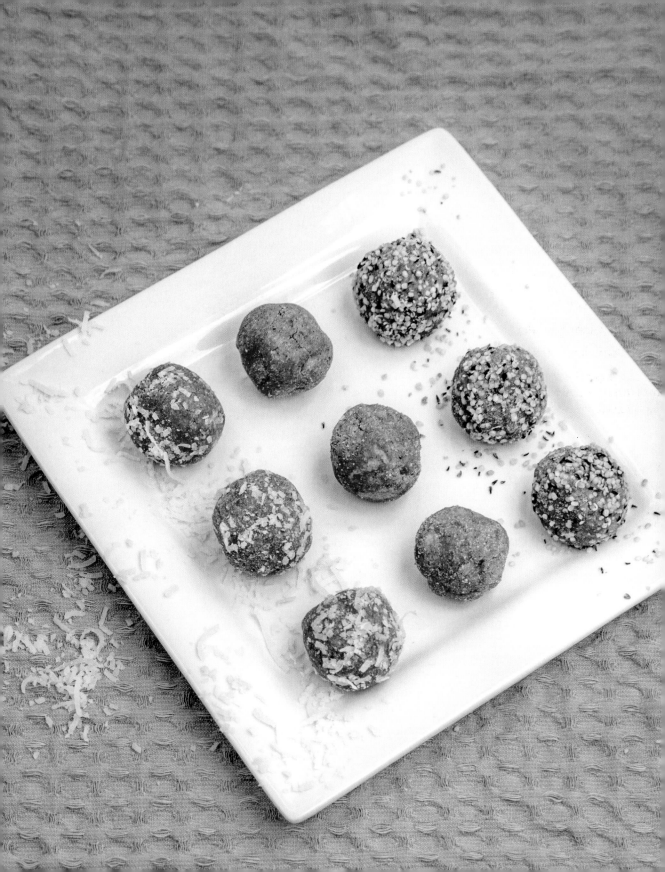

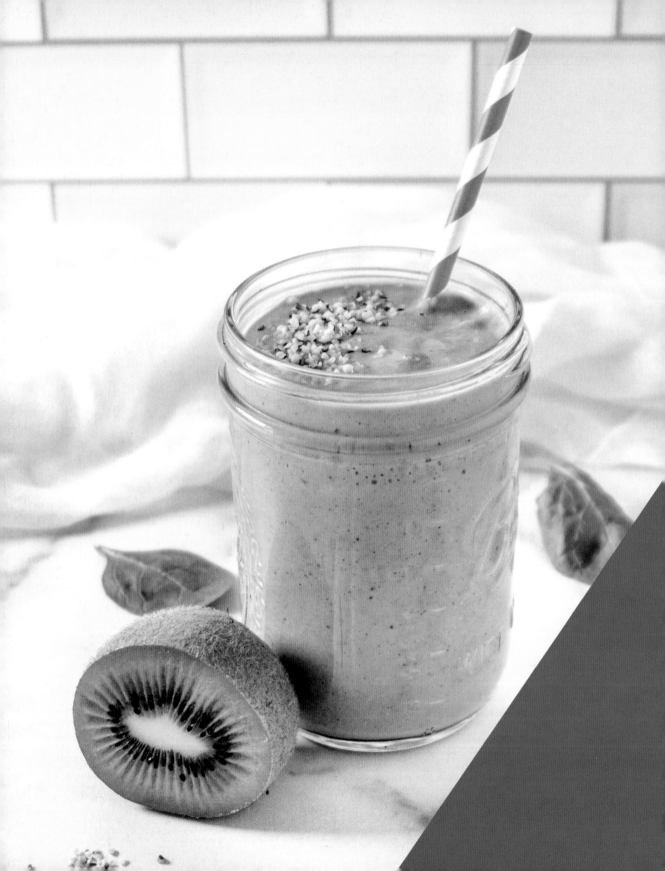

SMOOTHIES

Chocolate
MINT SMOOTHIE

YIELD: 1 serving
PREP TIME: 5 minutes
COOK TIME: —

1 cup unsweetened nondairy milk of choice

½ medium banana

½ cup baby spinach

¼ cup fresh mint leaves

2 tablespoons (1 scoop) collagen peptides or unflavored or chocolate-flavored protein powder

1 tablespoon cacao powder or cocoa powder

½ teaspoon ground cinnamon

1 ice cube

Put all the ingredients in a blender and blend until smooth.

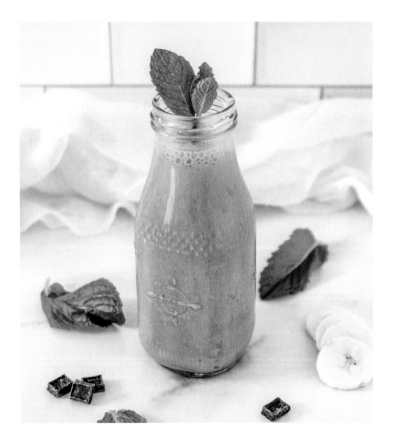

Sangria
SMOOTHIE

YIELD: 1 serving
PREP TIME: 5 minutes
COOK TIME: —

Put all the ingredients in a blender and blend until smooth.

½ cup pomegranate juice

½ cup water

½ medium orange, peeled and sectioned

¼ cup fresh or frozen raspberries

2 tablespoons (1 scoop) collagen peptides or unflavored or vanilla-flavored protein powder

1 tablespoon lime juice

1 teaspoon coconut oil

¼ teaspoon ground cinnamon

1 ice cube

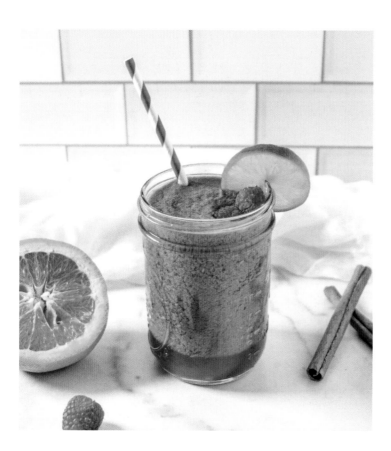

Citrus Boost
SMOOTHIE

YIELD: 1 serving
PREP TIME: 5 minutes
COOK TIME: —

¾ cup coconut water

½ medium orange, peeled and sectioned

¼ cup fresh or frozen mango chunks

¼ cup chopped carrots

¼ Hass avocado

2 tablespoons (1 scoop) collagen peptides or unflavored or vanilla-flavored protein powder

1 tablespoon ground flaxseed

¼ teaspoon ginger powder

¼ teaspoon turmeric powder

1 ice cube

Put all the ingredients in a blender and blend until smooth.

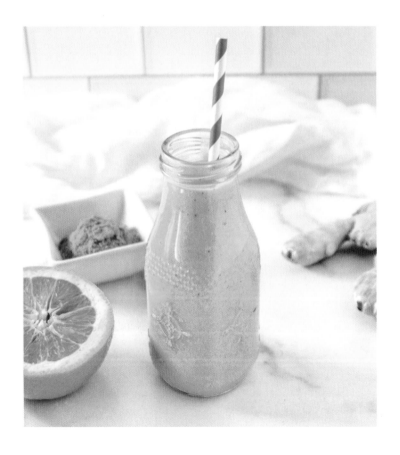

Can't Be Beet
SMOOTHIE

YIELD: 1 serving
PREP TIME: 5 minutes
COOK TIME: —

Put all the ingredients in a blender and blend until smooth.

¾ cup water

½ cup frozen blueberries

½ cup chopped baby kale

¼ cup chopped beets

2 tablespoons (1 scoop) collagen peptides or unflavored or vanilla-flavored protein powder

1 teaspoon coconut oil

¼ teaspoon ginger powder

1 ice cube

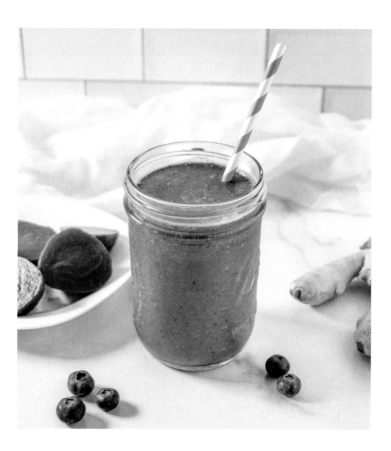

Green Pineapple
SMOOTHIE

YIELD: 1 serving
PREP TIME: 5 minutes
COOK TIME: —

1 cup unsweetened coconut milk

1 cup baby kale

½ cup fresh or frozen pineapple chunks

2 tablespoons (1 scoop) collagen peptides or unflavored protein powder

1 tablespoon ground flaxseed

1½ teaspoons coconut oil

½ teaspoon ginger powder

1 ice cube

Put all the ingredients in a blender and blend until smooth.

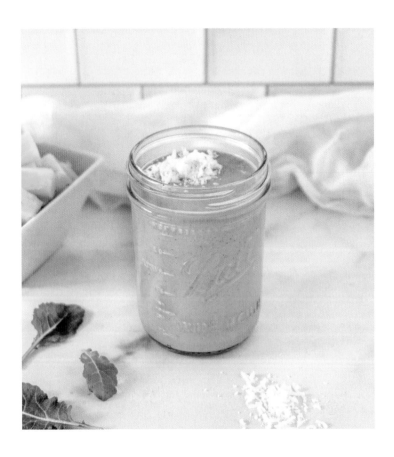

Skinny Monkey
SMOOTHIE

YIELD: 1 serving
PREP TIME: 5 minutes
COOK TIME: —

Put all the ingredients in a blender and blend until smooth.

1 cup unsweetened nondairy milk of choice

2 tablespoons (1 scoop) collagen peptides or unflavored or chocolate-flavored protein powder

½ medium banana

2 tablespoons chopped raw walnuts

1 tablespoon cacao powder or cocoa powder

1 tablespoon ground flaxseed

1 ice cube

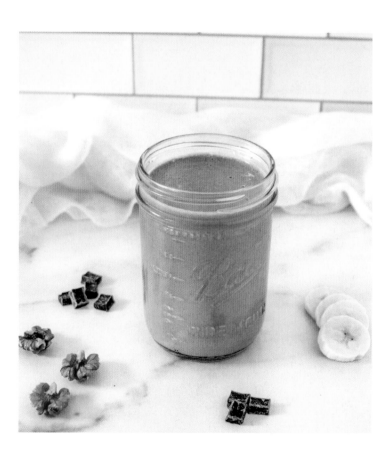

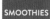

YIELD: 1 serving
PREP TIME: 5 minutes
COOK TIME: —

Matcha Power
SMOOTHIE

1 cup unsweetened nondairy milk of choice

1 kiwi, peeled

½ medium banana

½ cup baby spinach

¼ Hass avocado

2 tablespoons (1 scoop) collagen peptides or unflavored or vanilla-flavored protein powder

1 teaspoon hulled hemp seeds

1 teaspoon matcha powder

1 ice cube

Put all the ingredients in a blender and blend until smooth.

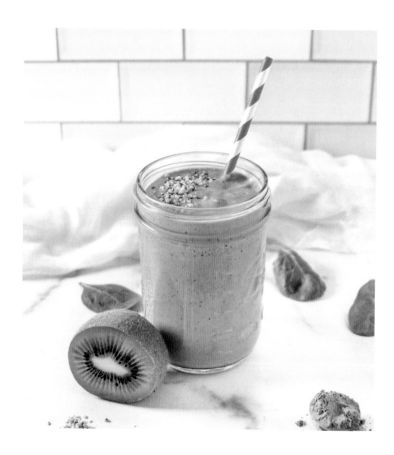

Strawberry Mint
SMOOTHIE

YIELD: 1 serving
PREP TIME: 5 minutes
COOK TIME: —

Put all the ingredients in a blender and blend until smooth.

¾ cup unsweetened nondairy milk of choice

½ cup full-fat plain Greek yogurt or nondairy yogurt

¾ cup fresh or frozen strawberries

¼ cup fresh mint leaves

2 tablespoons (1 scoop) collagen peptides or unflavored or vanilla-flavored protein powder

1 teaspoon chia seeds

1 ice cube

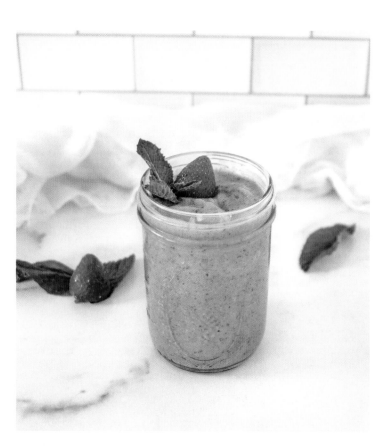

Anti-Inflammatory
SMOOTHIE

YIELD: 1 serving
PREP TIME: 5 minutes
COOK TIME: —

1 cup unsweetened nondairy milk of choice

½ cup fresh or frozen pineapple chunks

2 tablespoons (1 scoop) collagen peptides or unflavored protein powder

1 teaspoon avocado oil

1 teaspoon chia seeds

1 teaspoon turmeric powder

½ teaspoon ginger powder

Pinch of ground black pepper

Put all the ingredients in a blender and blend until smooth.

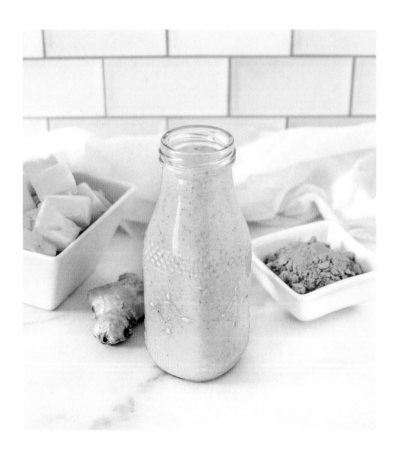

Blood Sugar Balancing
SMOOTHIE

YIELD: 1 serving
PREP TIME: 5 minutes
COOK TIME: —

Put all the ingredients in a blender and blend until smooth.

1 cup unsweetened nondairy milk of choice

2 tablespoons (1 scoop) collagen peptides or unflavored or vanilla-flavored protein powder

½ cup baby kale

½ cup frozen blueberries

¼ cup frozen cherries

1 tablespoon unsweetened almond butter

1 tablespoon ground flaxseed

1 teaspoon apple cider vinegar

½ teaspoon ground cinnamon

¼ teaspoon ginger powder

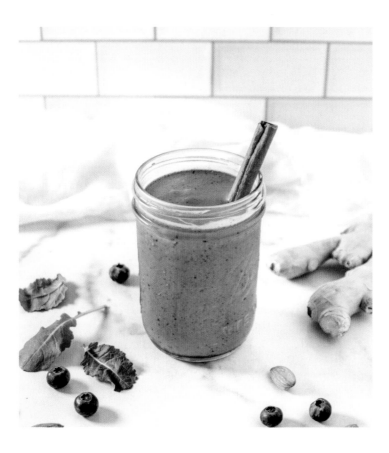

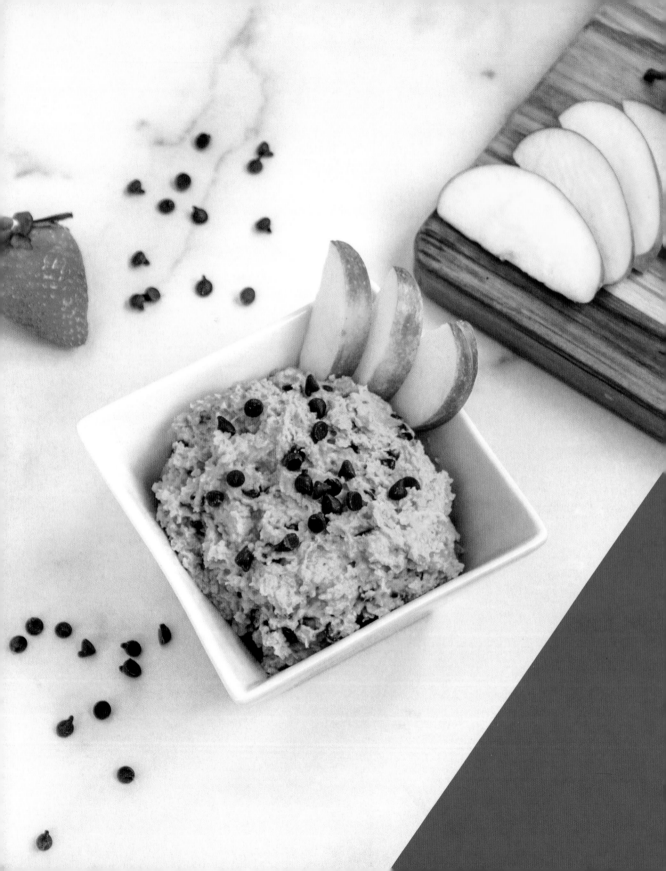

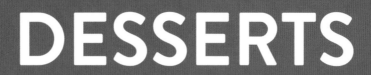

DESSERTS

Chocolate Sea Salt
BROWNIE BITES

YIELD: 12 balls

PREP TIME: 10 minutes, plus 1 hour to chill

COOK TIME: —

1 cup raw walnuts

1 cup pitted dates

¼ cup cacao powder or cocoa powder

2 tablespoons coconut oil, melted

1 tablespoon maple syrup

1 teaspoon vanilla extract

¼ cup dark chocolate chips

¼ teaspoon coarse sea salt

1. Put the walnuts, dates, cacao powder, melted coconut oil, maple syrup, and vanilla in a food processor and pulse until the walnuts are finely chopped and the mixture forms a sticky dough. Using your hands, roll the mixture into 12 balls, about 1 inch in diameter. Place the balls on a sheet pan lined with parchment paper or wax paper.

2. Put the chocolate chips in a small microwave-safe bowl and microwave for 30 seconds at a time, stirring after each increment, until melted.

3. Drizzle the melted chocolate over the balls and sprinkle with the salt.

4. Chill the balls for at least 1 hour before eating. Store in the refrigerator for up to 1 week.

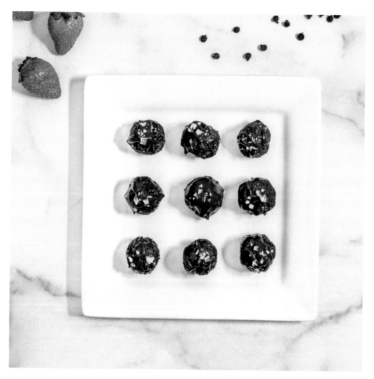

Avocado Key Lime
MOUSSE

YIELD: 2 servings
PREP TIME: 5 minutes, plus 1 hour to chill
COOK TIME: —

1. Zest the limes, setting aside the grated zest. Then juice the limes.

2. Put the avocados, lime juice, coconut milk, maple syrup, and vanilla in a food processor and process until smooth.

3. Divide the mousse between two serving cups and sprinkle with the lime zest. Chill the mousse for at least 1 hour before eating. Garnish each cup with 2 raspberries, if desired. Enjoy within 2 days.

2 Key limes

2 large Hass avocados, peeled and pitted

⅓ cup unsweetened coconut milk

1 tablespoon maple syrup

½ teaspoon vanilla extract

4 fresh raspberries, for garnish (optional)

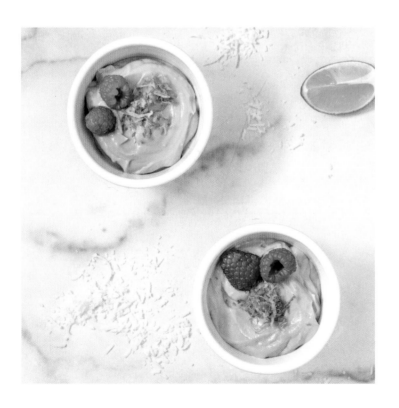

Summer
BERRY CRISP

YIELD: 4 servings
PREP TIME: 5 minutes
COOK TIME: 30 minutes

1 cup fresh or frozen
blackberries

1 cup fresh or frozen
blueberries

1 cup fresh or frozen
raspberries

1 cup fresh or frozen sliced
strawberries

1 cup blanched almond flour

½ cup chopped raw walnuts

¼ cup coconut oil, melted

2 tablespoons coconut sugar

1 teaspoon ground cinnamon

1. Preheat the oven to 400°F. Spray a 9-inch square baking pan with cooking spray.

2. Layer the berries in the prepared pan.

3. In a medium bowl, whisk together the almond flour, walnuts, coconut oil, coconut sugar, and cinnamon until crumbly. Sprinkle the crumb mixture on top of the berries.

4. Bake for 30 minutes, or until the topping is lightly browned and the berries are bubbling. Let cool slightly before serving.

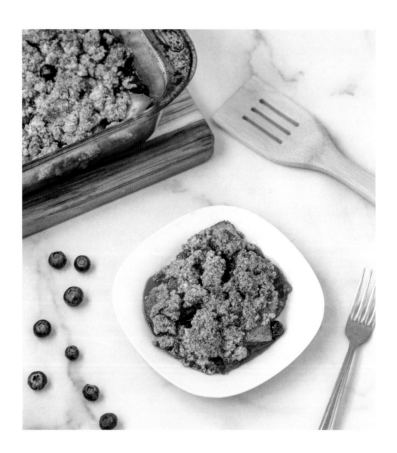

Chickpea
COOKIE BUTTER

YIELD: about 2 cups (¼ cup per serving)
PREP TIME: 5 minutes
COOK TIME: —

1. Put the chickpeas, cashew butter, maple syrup, flaxseed, vanilla, and salt in a food processor and process until smooth.

2. Remove the cookie butter from the food processor and stir in the chocolate chips.

3. Serve with the apple slices for dipping. Store in the refrigerator for up to 1 week.

1 (15-ounce) can chickpeas, drained and rinsed

½ cup cashew butter

1 tablespoon maple syrup

1 tablespoon ground flaxseed

2 teaspoons vanilla extract

Pinch of fine sea salt

½ cup dark chocolate chips

Sliced apples or other fruit of choice, for serving

YIELD: 12 truffles

PREP TIME: 10 minutes, plus
1 hour to chill

COOK TIME: —

Chocolate Mint
TRUFFLES

½ cup coconut flour

¼ cup unsweetened almond butter

¼ cup cacao powder or cocoa powder

1 tablespoon maple syrup

2 tablespoons coconut oil, melted

1 teaspoon peppermint extract

¼ cup dark chocolate chips

1. In a large bowl, thoroughly combine the coconut flour, almond butter, cacao powder, maple syrup, coconut oil, and peppermint extract. Using your hands, roll the mixture into 12 balls, about 1 inch in diameter.

2. Put the chocolate chips in a small microwave-safe bowl and microwave for 30 seconds at a time, stirring after each increment, until melted.

3. Use a toothpick to pick up a ball, dip it into the melted chocolate, and spin it around until completely covered. Tap the toothpick lightly against the side of the bowl so the excess chocolate drips off and the chocolate forms a thin layer around the ball. Place the chocolate-covered ball on a sheet pan lined with parchment paper or wax paper. Repeat with the remaining 11 balls.

4. Chill the truffles for at least 1 hour before eating. Store in the refrigerator for up to 1 week.

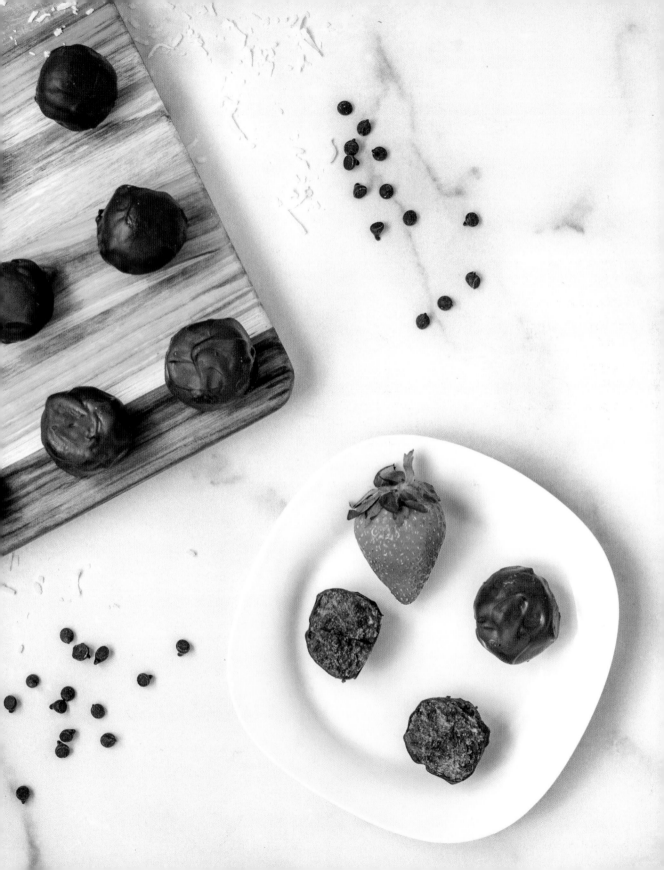

INDEX

ABOUT THE AUTHOR

Melissa Groves Azzaro, RDN, LD, is an integrative registered dietitian and the owner of Avocado Grove Nutrition & Wellness, an in-person and virtual private practice specializing in women's health and hormone issues, including PCOS and fertility. She uses a functional medicine, food-first approach that combines holistic lifestyle changes with evidence-based medicine.

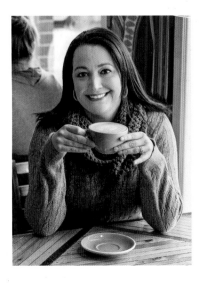

Melissa is a second-career dietitian, having worked as a copywriter and editor in medical advertising in New York for fifteen years before going back to school for nutrition. She has a BA in English and dance from Hofstra University and completed her BS in nutrition/dietetics and a dietetic internship at the University of New Hampshire.

She is a regular contributor to online magazines and food and nutrition blogs. She serves on the Dietitians in Integrative and Functional Medicine board as social media chair and on the New Hampshire state board as professional development chair. She is the recipient of the 2019 Emerging Professional in Women's Health Award and a recipient of a 2019 UpwaRD™ award given to up-and-coming dietitians in communications.

Melissa lives in Portsmouth, New Hampshire, with her husband and their four cats. She loves shopping at the farmers' market, hiking in the White Mountains, and breathing ocean air whenever possible.